OTHER BOOKS BY DR. GRANT

Growing Parents, Growing Children

The Caring Father

The Power of Affirming Touch

Questions Kids Ask About Sex

Living the Lord's Prayer Day by Day

ADHD
STRATEGIES FOR SUCCESS

How to Help the Child with ADHD

WILSON WAYNE GRANT, MD

iUniverse, Inc.
Bloomington

ADHD Strategies for Success
How to Help the Child with ADHD

iUniverse books may be ordered through booksellers or by contacting:

iUniverse
1663 Liberty Drive
Bloomington, IN 47403
www.iuniverse.com
1-800-Authors (1-800-288-4677)

ISBN: 978-1-4620-4240-1 (sc)
ISBN: 978-1-4620-4242-5 (hc)
ISBN: 978-1-4620-4241-8 (e)

Printed in the United States of America

iUniverse rev. date: 8/1/2011

Dedication

*To all the parents and
children who have shared with me
their struggles and successes
and thus have helped me understand the
Strategies for Success.*

CONTENTS

SECTION ONE
STRATEGIES IN DIAGNOSIS

CHAPTER ONE

*Questions You Have Always
Wanted to Ask, But ...!*

Questions and Answers

YOU have in your hand this book, *Strategies for Success*. I don't know why you picked it up. But it could be that you have questions like these:

> My six-year-old son's teacher has just told me that Jamie may need to be kept back in first grade. He has not learned to read. I never suspected a problem before. What should I do?

> My five-year-old is always into things. He can't seem to sit still, he can't pay attention to any activity for more than a few minutes, and he is always acting before he thinks. He is in trouble constantly. What have I done wrong?

> My nine-year-old has tried hard, but she has barely scraped by in school. She can answer questions orally, but when given tests or homework, she seldom finishes. When she does, she makes many errors. Maybe she's not as smart as I once thought.

I have tried everything, but Jimmy is still a difficult, unpredictable child. He is lovable but is getting into trouble all the time. Am I a failure as a parent?

My twelve-year-old is in the seventh grade. She has always passed in school, but each year has been a struggle. She seems bright and wants to learn. But she is poorly organized—she can't remember her assignments and forgets them when she does them. She starts out on a task with good intentions but is easily distracted. This year is tough. She just might fail.

None of these situations may match yours exactly, but I suspect you have many of the same feelings, hopes, frustrations, and questions shared by these parents.

Over the years, I have worked with thousands of parents and their children with behavior and learning problems. As I have sifted through their stories, I find one common thread: a string of unanswered questions.

This book, then, is about those questions. More importantly, it is about answers.

Strategies for Success grew out of frustration—mine and that of the many families with whom I have worked.

As a pediatrician and a specialist in child development, I spend much of my professional time working with children who are square pegs in round holes. Over the years, I have searched for a resource that would help parents (as well as teachers and other interested adults) understand their children with attention, learning, and behavior problems. Such a resource should also give them practical, usable tools with which to help their child succeed.

From the beginning, *Strategies for Success* has been designed to be a practical, honest, and readable guide. It gives parents a general understanding of why all children do not fit into the same mold and why some do not learn the same way as others. Concrete steps for seeking help are outlined. Then, in considerable detail, the book presents practical strategies for the day-to-day rearing of the "square peg."

This book does not try to push any one theory. Rather, it presents a balanced view of the facts as they are presently known. The methods developed here are tried and proven ones based on thorough research and the experiences of hundreds of parents and professionals. At each step, this book goes where you as a parent or teacher live and deals with those gut issues of importance to you, your child, and your family.

Universal Questions

When parents seek help, they have a mingling of hopes, concerns, and frustrations. From experience, I have learned that parents whose children are having any kind of difficulty are asking five basic questions.

These questions are not always stated openly, but they are there, at least subconsciously, waiting for answers.

These questions are:

1. *Is there anything wrong with my child?*

The desire of all parents for their children to be normal and healthy is universal and understandable. Our earliest dreams are of a child with no blemishes—physically, mentally, or emotionally. But of course, that perfect child exists only in our dreams.

As human beings, no child is perfect. In fact, all of us as humans are a mixture of strengths and weaknesses. There is a great deal of variation in development within all of us. These variations of development can at times cause concern. For example, Susan walked at nine months; Johnny didn't walk until thirteen months. Sammy learned to read in kindergarten; Mary is having trouble still—and she is in the middle of the first grade. Are these normal variations, or do they represent some kind of developmental abnormality?

These are common and legitimate questions parents ask. Sometimes all a parent needs is reassurance that, indeed, his or her child really is normal and there is no need to worry. At other times, parents know something is wrong, and they actually are asking, "What's wrong, and how bad is it?"

2. *What's wrong with my child?*

When their children are sick or disabled in any way, parents have a real need to know what the problem is. The more specific the diagnosis, the more satisfied they are. However, parents often go from place to place, professional to professional, and agency to agency without getting a specific answer.

Not long ago, I saw for the first time a twelve-year-old girl who had a significant reading problem. "What do you understand Kim's problem to be?" I asked.

"No one has ever told us," her mother replied. "I wish I knew." Kim's parents may have been given a diagnosis at some point in time, but they probably were not given one in terms they could understand and digest. Parents have a hard time complying with treatment or remedial programs when they have not been given a clear diagnosis or outline of the problem.

3. *What caused it?*

This is a most important question to parents. They have a natural need to know the cause of anything that hurts or hinders their children.

This intense need to know the cause is due to many factors. One that looms large is the universal tendency of parents to blame themselves for their children's problems. This is true whether their children have a simple cold ("I know I shouldn't have let him go out barefoot!") or something more serious, such as a birth defect. ("I've always wondered if it was my fault for not taking my vitamins regularly.") When anything happens to their children, parents immediately look to themselves.

They ask persistently, "What did I do wrong?" or "What should I have done that I didn't do?" (See the section on parental guilt in chapter 4.)

One of the things we try to do in this book is help parents see that multiple factors are involved in producing observed developmental problems, and seldom does the responsibility rest on the shoulders of the parents.

4. *What is my child's future?*

Besides guilt, concern over the child's future is the parent's most urgent worry. When possible, we will try to give parents a reliable appraisal of their children's future expectations. When we don't know, we will be honest.

I am wary of making specific long-range predictions: "He will never learn to read!" or "She will definitely go college." Children are amazingly resilient and have a way of making fools out of those who are too dogmatic about them. I try to express the attitude I call *optimistic realism*. This means being honest regarding the child's level of function at this point but having an open mind about the range of future possibilities.

5. *What can we do to help?*

This is a healthy, mature question. In the end, it is the most important one. When the parents are ready to ask this question, they can actively enter the therapeutic partnership with the child and others who might help. But they can only reach this point if the professional (doctor, teacher, psychologist, therapist) has honestly answered their questions about diagnosis, cause, and prognosis. Only then can they think creatively about solutions.

In one of my favorite *Peanuts* cartoons, Lucy, speaking to Charlie Brown, says, "There are no stupid questions. There are only stupid answers."

I agree. Parents should never be timid about asking questions to which they do not have the answers.

Success Breeds Success

Facing each of these questions as honestly and thoroughly as we can is our *Strategy for Success*.

Yes, success for your child—for his or her growth and your relationship with him or her—is the goal of this book. The children we focus on here have often met with failure after failure. Each failure tends to breed more failure until hope dies.

On the other hand, I firmly believe that success breeds success. Each success involves the child and the family in an upward spiral of future successes. Each success experienced by the child serves as a stepping stone to new ones.

Now on to success!

For Thought and Discussion

1. The five questions parents ask are listed below. Circle the ones for which you have not yet received satisfactory answers. Who might help you find the answers you seek?

a. Is there anything really wrong with my child?

b. If so, what is wrong?

c. What caused this problem?

d. What does this mean for my child's future?

e. What can we do to help?

2. Write out any additional questions you would like to discuss with a professional or other knowledgeable person.

3. Look through the table of contents of *Strategies for Success* and find chapters that you think may speak to your concerns.

CHAPTER TWO

"I've Tried Everything!"

The Variety of Attention and Learning Problems in Children: Mark

THE first time I saw Mark Wilson, he was balancing perilously on a waiting-room chair. He had already touched every toy in the room, inspected the receptionist's desk, and opened the bathroom door three times.

"Get down and be still, please," Mrs. Wilson commanded. She obviously had said this many times before.

Mark was placed in the custody of the office nurse, and I invited Mrs. Wilson into my office. Sighing, she plopped into a chair.

"I'm at the end of my rope with Mark," she began. "I've tried everything, but nothing works. I'm a failure." She paused, gathering her thoughts. "Sometimes I think I'm going out of my mind."

"Before we decide you're a failure," I interjected, "why don't you tell me more about Mark?"

Mrs. Wilson settled into the chair and concentrated on a spot in the ceiling.

"I really don't know where to begin. Mark is now eight, and he's failing the third grade in school. His teacher keeps telling me that he's intelligent, but he just doesn't seem to learn. He's in constant motion and can't pay attention to anything for more than a minute or two. He will finish an assignment only if the teacher stands right over him and continuously directs his attention to his work."

She continued quickly. "Actually, he has been a different child since birth. As an infant, he never had a very regular sleep pattern. He cried easily and frequently held his breath. But he seemed smart. He developed rapidly and he was walking, or rather running, by eleven months of age. By one year he was climbing on everything, but he fell all the time.

"By age three, his most outstanding characteristic was constant motion. But he never was mean. By being very strict with him at home, we usually could control him. But when he was away from home—like at the nursery or with sitters or neighbors—he would just get completely out of hand. He was not deliberately mean; it was as if he was following one impulse after another.

"His first-grade teacher loved him, but he frequently got into trouble. He was active, disruptive, and loud in class. He had difficulty staying in his seat, talked out of turn, and often didn't complete his assignments. His writing and coloring were messy. He was passed conditionally to the second grade." Mrs. Wilson paused to get her breath.

"Everyone hoped he would mature over the summer. But things weren't much better. He still couldn't read well. He had a short attention span and forgot his assignments. His relationship with other children deteriorated too. He so badly wanted to make friends, but friendships did not last long because of his bullying and impulsive behavior. Now, in the third grade, he really is behind. Everyone keeps saying he is smart, but his reading is poor and he just can't get organized."

Mrs. Wilson sighed again. "That's it," she said. "Now we are here."

From my experience working with other children like Mark, I realized that here was a mother who deserved a medal for endurance, patience, and care.

When Mark first entered my office, he was somewhat subdued and quiet. He watched me carefully. He responded quickly to my questions. But soon he began to answer my questions before I finished with irrelevant questions of his own. My examination revealed no signs of physical illness. His motor coordination was somewhat immature for his age. For instance, Mark could not stand on one foot for more than five seconds. His writing was messy and disorganized.

I then read the following report sent to me by Mark's present teacher:

> Mark is repeatedly tardy coming in from the playground at noon and at PE. The coach has complained to me several times about having to tell Mark over and over to line up when the bell rings to come in. He doesn't respond when I give group directions to get coats—even to go home—making it necessary for me to give him individual directions.
>
> Mark is capable of successfully doing all third-grade work. He retains his vocabulary very well. His phonics knowledge is above average, and he is one of my fastest students in number combination drills. He earned a straight one hundred on his spelling words when I let him answer them orally. But on the same words written at his desk, he got only sixty.

Earlier, Dr. Waters, the staff psychologist, had administered a variety of intelligence, achievement, and personality tests to Mark. Interestingly, his IQ was 116—well above average. He obviously was not stupid. This score contrasted dramatically with his failing grades in school.

Dr. Waters also commented, "Mark has an extremely short attention span." On tests of reading skills, he was behind his age level. He had particular difficulty in recognizing and sounding out words. His reading ability was on a first-grade level. Dr. Waters also commented that Mark seemed to have a great deal of difficulty in organizing himself and got mixed up when a series of instructions were given to him.

Pieces of a Puzzle

Mrs. Wilson's detailed history of Mark's past, my own examination, and the report from the psychologist and teacher began to fall into place like the scattered pieces of a puzzle.

As I put the data together, Mark's behavior and achievement fell into a recognizable pattern: Mark is a typical (if extreme) example of what has been commonly called *the hyperactive child*. He has what is today called Attention Deficit/Hyperactivity Disorder or ADHD.

Anyone in daily contact with Mark quickly realized that something is out of order with him. His difficulty in settling into most any environment made him a square peg in a round hole. This condition led to conflict and frustration at home, underachievement at school, and poor relationships on the playground.

Another End of the Spectrum: Karen

All children with learning and attention problems are not as obviously different as Mark. He represents one end of a spectrum—the more demonstratively active child.

At the other end of this spectrum is Karen. As a preschooler, Karen was a likeable child but was talkative and aggressive. Her social behavior, however, did not appear all that unusual.

The first sign of difficulty was noted by her kindergarten teacher, who reported that she had a short attention span, particularly when working in groups and when performing seat work. She was easily distracted and often did not complete assigned tasks. She was a pleasant, cooperative child who was not a behavior problem. Now she was in first grade and could read in small groups, but her seat work was messy and incomplete, with many inconsistent errors. Her teacher reported to her parents toward the middle of the school year: "Karen seems quite smart, and she is sweet. But she just doesn't get her work done. She is really not working up to her potential."

Karen, too, had been tested by a psychologist. She scored above average on the intelligence test, and the achievement tests showed that she had learned the material expected for first grade. However, while being tested, Karen was easily distracted and often responded impulsively, making frequent careless errors. Her writing was messy and irregular, and she had difficulty organizing material on the page.

In retrospect, her parents noted that she could not concentrate as well as her brothers on games, TV, or family activities. While she wanted to be cooperative with home activities and chores, she required repeated directions and frequent reminders. Her room was messy, and she had trouble finding things.

To the casual observer, Karen's behavior and performance seemed pretty normal. But in subtle ways, she shared many characteristics with Mark, particularly in the inability to control and focus her attention. She represents the other end of the spectrum of the child with attention problems—the child with attention problems but without significant hyperactivity or impulsiveness.

There is no one stereotypical picture of this common disorder. Between the extremes of Mark and Karen a spectrum of children exists who share, to a greater or lesser degree, a pattern of neuro-developmental dysfunction that results in problems for them, their parents, their teachers, and their friends. Karen had subtle symptoms, was less disruptive, and showed primarily performance lag. On the other hand, Mark had obvious symptoms, was often disruptive, and had performance and behavior problems most of them time.

In a real sense, Karen and Mark were *square pegs in round holes.* Children like them don't easily fit in the boxes life throws at them.

In the next chapter, we will discuss in detail what makes Mark and Karen different from other children and explore the common denominators underlying their development.

For Thought and Discussion

1. Do you have, or know of, a child like Mark or Karen? List below characteristics your child has in common with Mark or Karen. Also list some characteristics in which your child is not like Mark or Karen:

Characteristics in common:

Mark

Karen

Characteristics that are different:

Mark

Karen

2. Now look at the children described at the beginning of chapter 1. Do any of them seem more like your child? Think about it. Discuss

CHAPTER THREE

Three-Ring Circus—Defining Attention Deficit Disorder

Real but Misunderstood

CHILDREN may have difficulty in learning and behavior control for many reasons. Mark and Karen, on the surface, appear quite different. But they share much in common. Their problems are due to one of the most common childhood developmental problem—Attention Deficit/ Hyperactivity Disorder.

The existence of a syndrome characterized by varying degrees of short attention span, impulsiveness, disorganization, and physical hyperactivity has been recognized since the early 1900s. For years parents, educators, and physicians talked about the "hyperactive child." As revealed in our discussion of Mark and Karen, however, the hyperactive child is only one end of a long and varied spectrum. Thanks to many years of ongoing research, we now have a better understanding of the many different patterns presented by children with attention deficits and related problems.

This neuro-behavioral disorder is one of the most widely studied conditions of children. Thousands of research reports have been published in a wide variety of professional journals as well as many articles in popular magazines. Yet this condition remains one of the most misunderstood and debated developmental disorders of children. I hope this book will help clarify this confusion for parents and teachers.

The condition we now call Attention Deficit/Hyperactivity Disorder is not new. It is a condition that has affected children for all of human history. It is only in the last century, however, that clinicians have described in systematic fashion children who failed to achieve and adjust due to problems with attention and focus.

Over the years the names used to describe this developmental disorder have evolved. Commonly used at one time or the other are terms such as *cerebral dysfunction, hyperactivity disorder, hyperactivity, impulse control dysfunction, attention deficit disorder (ADD), etc.*

Today the term *attention deficit disorder (ADD)* is often used to refer to children with attention problems without hyperactivity. *Attention deficit hyperactivity disorder (ADHD)* is frequently used to refer to children with attention problems along with hyperactivity and impulsiveness. However, these terms are often used interchangeably, for they simply represent differing views of the same condition.

Definition of Attention Deficit/ Hyperactivity Disorder

Attention Deficit Disorder is circumscribed by three primary developmental characteristics:

- Disordered Attention Control
- Disordered Impulse Control
- Disordered Activity Control

Now let us look at each of these in detail to see how they are reflected in a child's learning and behavior patterns. The more we understand, the more we can help.

Disordered Attention Control

The most common observation of parents and teachers is, "He has a short attention span," or "She can't concentrate on her work."

Indeed, children with attention deficit have an inability to control and modulate their attention. To a greater or lesser degree, they have trouble focusing their attention on a specific task or activity for an appropriate length of time. Observing them, it appears their minds are bouncing from one interest to another with rapidity and lack of order.

The inability to focus and concentrate appropriately for their age is a function of their neurological immaturity. These children have varying levels of difficulty in handling and organizing their sensory input.

When engaged in any activity, one's body is constantly bombarded with a myriad of stimuli. External stimuli flood the nervous system via all the senses: through vision, hearing, touch, and smell. Added to this are internal stimuli, such as muscle and joint sensation, known as kinesthetic sense (i.e., leg cramps), internal organ sensation (i.e., sensation of hunger or a full bladder), and emotional sensations (i.e., sadness, anger, joy, and excitement). All of these stimuli are bombarding the senses continuously.

Normally one is not aware of all, or even most, of these sensations. The human brain has the ability to screen out the irrelevant and unimportant in order to focus on the few that are relevant to one's intentions at the time.

When someone is reading a book, he focuses on the visual stimulus of the words and the images in the mind. He mentally ignores the many other stimuli. He does not hear the noise of the air conditioner fan or the quiet chatter of the children. He is not aware of the pressure of the chair on the buttocks. He even screens out for the moment internal feelings of sadness, worry, or joy. He is by this process "concentrating."

Now after he sits for a while in one position, he may get a cramp in a leg, and the pain will be significant enough to arouse him from his concentration on the book so that he will change position. If the doorbell rings, he shifts his attention to that stimulus, or a full bladder may arouse him to get up and go to the bathroom. But for the most part, he is oblivious to most stimuli impinging on the body. That is concentration. One's power of concentration in a given situation is a function of:

(1) the person's ability to attend or tune into the significant stimulus;

(2) the strength of the stimulus for that person (how important it is to the individual);

(3) and the presence of distractions in the environment.

With most people, the ability to concentrate is variable. Some simply have longer, more powerful attention spans than others. The nature of the stimulus is important. What is of interest to one person will not necessarily appeal to another. One person can sit for hours reading a novel, another listening to music, still another working a complicated puzzle. To others, any of these activities lose their appeal quickly. They become distracted and look for other things to do. The more distractions present, the more difficult it is to focus on the important stimulus. Attention span also varies with age. Infants and preschoolers have fairly short attention spans, usually measured in minutes for most activities. By kindergarten age, the attention span has increased significantly. By early adolescence, attention abilities on the average reach adult levels.

The child with ADHD is not able to maintain sustained attention as well, or as long, as the average child his or her age. In fact, more than anything else, poor quality of attention sets him apart from his peers. He cannot effectively screen the many stimuli, relevant and irrelevant, surrounding him. Instead, he is trying to attend to all of these stimuli at the same time. To a greater or lesser degree, he is at the mercy of every passing sight, sound, touch, mood, or internal sensation. He cannot effectively screen out extraneous stimuli in order to focus on the appropriate ones. Only a very strong stimulus (an activity or object of greater interest to him) can override all the others and capture the child's individual attention.

In the classroom setting, the child with normal concentration focuses on the teacher and hears his assignment. The child with attention problems turns to the teacher with the intention of getting the assignment. But soon he hears the faint sounds of a car passing in the street; his eyes are caught by the sunlight reflecting off the window; he feels his shoes pressing his big toe; he senses the first growls of hunger emanating from his stomach. Because of his inability to screen out or ignore any of the stimuli, his attention is diverted from one to the other. He thus misses the instructions for the test, gets started late, or does not finish. He will likely make inconsistent, careless errors in material he otherwise knows well. The result is another poor grade.

Otherwise bright, alert children may do poor academic work in school simply because they cannot focus their attention on a task long enough to complete it. In addition, the quality of their work is poor because of inefficiency, carelessness, and inadequate self-monitoring for errors.

Disordered Impulse Control

"Jenny is always acting before she thinks," one mother remarked. This is an apt description of the child with impulse control problems. Researcher Virginia Douglas[1] pointed out years ago that children with attention deficit have an inability *to stop, look, and listen*. They make decisions and act before all the data is in. They stop listening before they have heard the entire question. They plunge ahead on orders from their impulses without stopping to evaluate the consequences of their acts. This impulsiveness can be observed in several areas of behavior.

Physical Activity—The non-goal-directed, disorganized activity is often the result of following one impulse after another without evaluating the consequences of the acts.

Speech—Impulsive children are likely to speak whatever enters their minds at the moment without evaluating whether their words are timely or appropriate. They may speak loudly, interrupt often, and ask irrelevant, even embarrassing questions. In most of these cases, the children seem unaware of the inappropriateness of their responses; they likely will genuinely regret what they have done as soon as they have done it.

Social Relationships—They may push, hit, or shove playmates, not maliciously, but impulsively, without thinking or evaluating the effects on others. They tend to shift the tempo and substance of play, putting themselves out of step with their playmates and creating friction. This impulsiveness creates problems in controlling the intensity of emotional

---

1   Douglas, Virginia, "Stop, Look and Listen: The Problem of Sustained Attention an Impulse Control," *Canadian Journal of Behavioral Sciences*, Vol. 4, No. 4, 1972.

reactions. The emotional tone tends to oscillate from excitement to frustration, or from happiness to sadness, quickly and for little reason.

Task Performance—Impulsive children tend to make careless errors on tasks requiring continuous performance or frequent decision making. They tend to respond with the first idea that comes into their minds without stopping to evaluate whether it is appropriate. For instance, they often make many errors on written spelling tests even though they have previously shown they know the words.

Disordered Activity Control

The very term "hyperactivity" is derived from the long-standing observations that certain children exhibit a degree, and kind, of physical activity that sets them apart from other children their age. That is why the label "hyperactive" has stuck.

In the more obvious cases, hyperactive children are restless, incessantly going from one activity to another. At play they tend to be loud and boisterous, constantly changing activities and disrupting the play of other children. In the classroom, they get up and down, wiggle in their chairs, and even walk about the room. Most tasks are accomplished with an excess of body movement—much of it irrelevant to the task at hand. They run when they should be walking and talk when they should be listening. They crave attention and praise but always seem to be doing those things that get them into trouble.

Thus, they do appear hyperactive—that is, to have increased activity. But in reality, the problem is not so much increased activity as disorganized and unstructured activity. Researchers have placed a modified pedometer, a watch-like instrument that measures body movement, on children with and without hyperactivity. Surprisingly, in such experiments children with hyperactivity do not necessarily move substantially more than other children.

However, hyperactive children have a different *quality* to their movement. They have an excess of random, disorganized, and non-goal-directed body movement. Those of us who have worked with these children for a long time realize that it is the quality, not necessarily the quantity, of body movement that interferes with their adjustment to life's demands.

The random and disorganized nature of the activity does, however, give the appearance of increased body movement. It is this disruptive bodily activity that is most easily noticed by parents, teachers, and casual observers. Although the most easily noticed of the symptoms, the body activity is not always most important.

A Common Thread

Is there a common thread that ties these developmental dysfunctions together?

Indeed, there is.

Common to all of these disruptive symptoms is a lack of organization and control. It is as if a traffic light at a very busy intersection has gone awry, directing the traffic in a random and disorganized manner—sending the vehicles off in all directions at the same time. And in fact, something like that is what is happening in the child's brain.

Underlying the poor control of activity, attention, and impulse is a dysfunction of the interior of the brain resulting in less than normal mental organization. That part of the brain responsible for organizing, sequencing, and controlling mental activity is simply not working on a level appropriate for the child's age. This underlying disorganization in mental function leads to a general disorganized approach to tasks and the poorly controlled expression of activity, attention, and impulse.

Furthermore, evidence is accumulating that suggests this mental disorganization results from a combination of biochemical abnormalities within certain portions of the brain. A group of chemicals, called neuro-transmitters, are present in minute quantities within the brain. Their function is to facilitate the transmission of nerve impulses from one brain cell to another.

Data derived from various studies indicate that the balance of these neuro-transmitters differs in a subtle way in individuals with ADHD when compared with others. Thus the poor mental organization is a physical—some would say a neurological—disorder, not simply an emotional adjustment problem.

This imbalance in the neuro-transmitters affects performance and behavior in a variety of ways. All children with ADHD do not experience the same problems when confronted with a task, but any given child will likely demonstrate some combination of these difficulties:

- Short attention span
- Distractibility
- Slow reaction time
- Delayed motor speed
- Difficulty in interpreting and responding to cues from other people and the environment (trouble interpreting what people mean by the tone of their voice, facial expressions, etc.)
- Slower response to reinforcement (to discipline)
- Rapid mood changes, with poor control of feelings
- Poor self-monitoring (they are not able to stop, look, and listen or to anticipate the consequences of their actions)

Every Child Is Different

It helps to visualize the spectrum of ADHD as three overlapping circles: one circle represents focused attention, one circle represents impulsiveness, and one circle represents hyperactivity. These different behavioral symptoms overlap to varying patterns—and degrees. Subtle shades of differences exist. While many children will express all of these dysfunctions in an observable manner, other children will express only one or two of these developmental symptoms.

The truly hyperactive child will be noticed early, because he disrupts everyone. In other children, the impulsiveness will stand out. Then there are children with a subtle attention deficit but little hyperactivity or impulsiveness who go unnoticed most of the time. But such a child, like Karen in the previous chapter, may suffer just as much.

Children vary widely in the degree or intensity of involvement. Some will have only mild degrees of the developmental dysfunctions and cope adequately in most situations and decompensate only at times and places of increased demand and stress. In others, all three circles overlap, and they have severe involvement in all areas and can hardly cope under any circumstances. There are no stereotypes.

A child like Mark, whom we met in the previous chapter, has *Attention Deficit with Hyperactivity (ADHD)*. He has every symptom listed to some degree: inattention, impulsiveness, and hyperactivity—all three circles overlap. Karen, on the other hand, represents a child with *Attention Deficit without hyperactivity (ADD)*. Her primary problem is inattention and disorganization. As mentioned earlier, Mark and Karen represent a difference in quantity of expression rather than a difference in quality of expression of the underlying neuro-developmental dysfunction. Her circle of inattention does not overlap substantially with the one of hyperactivity or impulsiveness.

The Life Cycle of the Child with ADHD

A typical characteristic of ADD or ADHD is the presence of the functional problems from an early age. However, the differences may be quite subtle, to the point of not being noticed by parents or teachers during the preschool years in the child with mild or moderate involvement. The child with more significant hyperactivity and impulsiveness, however, will stand out, even at this age.

Although toddlers are naturally very active, distractible, and impulsive, a hyperactive child at this age tends to be more restless, uncontrollable, and less responsive to discipline than the average toddler. He may have more temper tantrums and accidents. Except in extreme cases, however, it is very difficult for even the best clinician to differentiate between the normal and hyperactive toddler.

Thus the typical character of Attention Deficit Disorder may not be clearly discernible until the child begins kindergarten or first grade. While the normal preschooler is outgrowing the overactivity of toddlerhood, the child with ADHD stands out in the crowd, exhibiting to varying degrees hyperactivity, distractibility, impulsiveness, and emotional variability. The difference between him and his peers becomes quite obvious to most observers, particularly to those who must live with him. His inability to respond to discipline, cooperate in groups, and work up to his intellectual potential leads parents and teachers to ask, "What is wrong?"

On the other hand, the mildly involved child may appear fairly normal most of the time but exhibits easy distractibility, short attention span, and inefficiency in learning tasks. Karen from chapter 2 is a good example.

Without treatment, attention deficits continue to interfere with the child's life throughout the elementary school years—sometimes seemingly worse as the child continues to fall behind his peers in maturity and performance.

Near the time of puberty, the hyperactivity and impulsiveness tend to improve. Symptoms of inattention and disorganization are more likely to persist into adolescence and adulthood. As researchers have been able to observe individuals with attention deficit grow into adulthood, it is apparent that some symptoms do persist. But for most people, their dysfunctions improve progressively through puberty and adolescence. (Later in the book we will delve more deeply into what happens to children with ADHD as they become adolescents and adults.)

As we will see in the next chapter, early recognition and comprehensive management will help children overcome their hurdles in learning and progress toward success and achievement.

The Relationship of ADHD to Other Learning Disabilities

You may have noticed that there is one aspect of Mark's behavior that we have not mentioned. In addition to the typical characteristics of attention deficit and hyperactivity we have just discussed, Mark had some other problems. In school he was slow in learning to read, and on the psycho-educational tests given to him, he had significant perceptual-motor problems, language delay, and poor spelling.

These cognitive difficulties pointed toward Mark having a Specific Learning Disability. This is a condition in which there is interference in the child's ability to take in, assimilate, and recall information.

A specific learning disability may exist alone or may occur in association with various degrees of attention deficit and hyperactivity.

Not all hyperactive children have learning disabilities, and not all learning-disabled children have ADHD. But these developmental disorders do frequently overlap. A further discussion of the various types of learning disabilities will be found in chapter 12.

For Thought and Discussion

1. Look over the description of ADHD in this chapter. Grade your child on these characteristics:

   Disordered activity control: mild, moderate, severe
   Disordered attention control: mild, moderate, severe
   Disordered impulse control: mild, moderate, severe

2. As discussed in this chapter, these primary developmental disorders may lead to a combination of functional and behavioral problems, such as:

   Short attention span
   Distractibility
   Slow reaction time
   Delayed motor speed
   Difficulty in responding to cues from others
   Slow response to discipline
   Rapid mood changes
   Poor self-monitoring
   Overexcitability
   Difficulty sequencing (putting things in order)

   Look over this list. Circle the ones that apply to your child.

3. What problems other than the ones circled are you concerned about?

4. What is the number one problem you are having with your child and for which you would like help?

Thinking through this worksheet carefully and taking time to mull it over will be of great help. The more you can focus on the core problem, the more effective you will be in management.

SECTION TWO
STRATEGIES IN MANAGEMENT

Chapter Four

Directions to Success

The Most Important Step

"What can be done to help my child?"

This question is one for which parents urgently seek answers. It is the question to which all others should lead. The following chapters squarely face this question, with the intention of giving some practical, useful answers to the pivotal question.

Up to this point, we have learned many things about children who have attention deficits and related problems. We have learned that children with Attention Deficit/Hyperactivity Disorder have three major areas of dysfunction:

- Disordered attention control
- Disordered activity control
- Disordered impulse control

These dysfunctions result in a mixed bag of behaviors that, to varying degrees, affect the child's ability to adjust, learn, and relate. Some of these behaviors are:

- Short attention span
- Distractibility
- Slowed reaction time

- Delayed motor speed
- Poor response to reinforcement (i.e., difficult to discipline)
- Rapid mood changes with poor control of emotional expression
- Poor self-monitoring
- Inability to stop, look, and listen before acting
- Inefficiency in sequencing, patterning, and organizing their actions

We also have learned that these children are not all alike. They come in a variety of packages. They do not all have the same behavior repertoire. The eventual behavior the child exhibits at home, in the classroom, and on the playground is a product of many forces that combine to mold the child's behavior.

Some children have minimal hyperactivity, attention deficit, and impulsiveness. Their daily life is not noticeably affected except at times, and points, of demand and stress. Others are more totally involved and have problems with adjustment and achievement at every turn. Success in most all things eludes them.

Whatever shape your child's behavior and performance takes, whatever his or her pattern of behavior, the basic principles of management are pretty much the same, with some variation to meet specific needs. We hope to provide strategies useful to all, while at the same time providing specific strategies for specific problems.

Five Basic Steps

There are five basic steps to success:

1. The first step is to understand. The people closest to the child (parents, teachers, and other significant adults in his or her life) need to gain an understanding of the nature and reasons for the child's bothersome and unproductive behavior. This involves coming to accept the truth that *this is a child with a problem—not a problem child.* This understanding, in itself, is therapeutic. By knowing the why of the child's behavior, parents and teachers can react innately in a supportive and remedial way. It is this kind of information that the earlier chapters of this book attempt to provide.

2. Search for and remove (or treat) any causative or aggravating factors when possible. This step will be discussed in the next chapter.

3. Provide a structured, organized, supportive environmental cocoon. Methods that help one to do this effectively will be discussed at length throughout the rest of this book.

4. Provide an appropriate educational environment in which the child's unique developmental needs are addressed. This will be discussed in chapters 13 and 14.

5. Consider the wise and careful use of medication when indicated. This will be discussed in chapter 7.

How to Take These Steps

To carry out this treatment plan effectively, the following methods will be needed:

1. Parent and family orientation. That is what this book is all about. *Strategies for Success* orients parents and other interested parties to the developmental reasons behind the child's problems and provides a step-by-step guide to parents.

2. Medical evaluation and follow up. A physician who is knowledgeable in the field of pediatrics, child development, psychiatry, or neurology will help assess the child's strength and weaknesses, counsel the parents in the necessary steps, point them to other helpful professionals, and supervise medical therapy when needed.

3. Educational intervention. Most children with attention deficits and related learning disabilities will usually have specific educational needs—needs that will require varying levels of evaluation and individualized instruction and/or classroom modification.

4. Behavioral therapy. In this book, we present the primary behavioral structure needed to help the child with ADHD function more normally. However, many of these children, as well as their families, will benefit from a formal program of behavior modification supervised by a psychologist or other trained professional.

5. Family counseling. Some level of counseling for the family and child will often help in dealing with the distorted family relationships brought on by the child's behavior. Individual as well as group counseling may be useful. Some families will have innate skills that will facilitate their coping without any formal outside counseling. Others will need short-term, straightforward behavior management advice. Others will need more extensive help in dealing not only with behavioral management issues but also with deeper emotional issues that affect family relationships.

Management: Not Cure or Treatment!

In *Strategies for Success,* we repeatedly talk about *management* of Attention Deficit Disorder. Given our current state of knowledge, there is no such thing as a cure of ADHD. There are various forms of treatment. However, the goal of treatment is to put in the hands of parents and eventually the children tools that facilitate their own management of their life.

"Management" in this manner is necessary because current knowledge tells us that attention-deficit/hyperactivity disorder, in all of its forms, is a lifelong condition. Its status changes over time as the individual progresses through sequential stages of development, with a decrease in intensity but not elimination of the underlying symptoms. Thus life success is proportional to success in "managing" the functional disruptions of ADHD.

The Eventual Goal

The eventual goal is to help children with ADHD grow into adolescents and adults who can manage their own ADHD. To do this, they will need to walk for themselves the same steps we have already mapped for the parents:

They need to learn the basic facts of ADHD. This helps them to understand why they do things the way they do. This comes by learning all they want to know—and at times more than they want to know— about the physiology and psychology of ADHD. For most individuals, this knowledge is acquired gradually and not before the teen years.

Some may be into the late teens or early adulthood before they are ready to deal with neuropsychology as it applies to them.

They need to learn how to manage the dysfunctions that persist and interfere with their performance and well-being. For instance, they will need to learn how to deliberately sequence and organize day-to-day work. They will need to develop conscious methods of impulse control. They certainly will need to learn how to screen out distractions and focus on the significant task.

They will need to take responsibility for the external help they may need, such as taking medication or seeking psychological consultation.

They will need to accept themselves as they are with all their unique strengths and weaknesses. This final step depends a great deal on the degree of success they experience in school and in interpersonal relationships

There Is Hope and Help

From my years of working with children, I know there are no magic, easy, once-and-for-all solutions to the behavior and academic problems of these children.

It is necessary to take all five of the steps outlined in this chapter and be prepared to work over the long haul. If we do, we can see immediate, positive results and can be assured of long-term, ongoing success as well. My experience over time shows that untreated children have an increased chance of growing into adults with many personal, social, and work problems.

However—and this is an important however—many other studies show that when such children receive the comprehensive treatment we are talking about here, involving all five steps, their chances of growing into healthy adults with minimal adjustment problems are very great. The rest of this book presents a comprehensive treatment strategy in which parents, teachers, and other caring professionals work together to obtain success for the child.

As the child works through these steps, he will be coming to the point where he can successfully manage his ADHD himself. His parents' job will then be that of cheerleaders.

I can remember a time when we talked about children "outgrowing" their hyperactivity and attention problems. This belief was based in part on wishful thinking. But there was the real observation that with advancing age, many of the bothersome symptoms did seem to go away or get better. As researchers have studied a large number of children with ADHD into adulthood over the past two decades, we now know that it is essentially a lifelong condition.

However, dramatic changes (largely for the better) do occur. Yes, there is a definite pattern of progressive improvement in all of the behavioral symptoms of ADHD from early childhood through puberty to adulthood. This improvement is slow but steady through the elementary school years; often accelerates during the pubertal years of middle school; continues to slowly improve during the later teen years; and levels off during early adulthood.

The most dramatic change occurs in the behavioral symptoms of hyperactivity, impulsiveness, and emotional control prior to puberty. There is less dramatic change in disorders of organization, sequencing, and attention. Two or three decades ago, the focus of parents, teachers, and clinicians was more on the hyperactivity and impulsiveness. Thus, we had the impression that children "grew out of" their condition. We now know that the more significant organizational and attention problems are likely to persist, to varying degrees, into the teen and adult years.

Reasons for Positive Change

Most children with ADHD grow into adults who are well-adjusted and successful. Two processes account for the overall healthy outlook for children diagnosed and treated for ADHD.

Physical Maturation

First, biology is on their side. Research points to ADHD being caused by dysfunctions in certain portions of the brain. In fact, the problem very well may be disordered communication between different areas of the brain and its organizational, or control, center.

The human nervous system is incompletely developed at birth. While all the nerve cells and fibers are in place, they are not insulated from each other by the natural nerve insulator, myelin. From birth onward, a process of "myelination" occurs. Slowly, but inevitably, myelin is deposited about the nerves in the brain and spinal cord. As this happens more and more, circuits come into action that allow more neurological function. Therefore, we observe the natural progression of child development in which motor skills, speech, and reasoning progressively develop with each day, week, month, and year of growth.

While the bulk of myelination occurs during the early years, this process continues right up to puberty. During the elementary school years, new circuits are becoming available to the brain's "computer." This allows the brain to find additional ways of doing its many of tasks.

This process of physical maturation in the central nervous system provides the brain with the opportunity to use alternate pathways for those that may not be working up to capacity.

Learning

Another very important process is going on at the same time physical maturation is occurring. Learning is happening. The child learns over time how to compensate for the various functional disabilities. This process is essentially unconscious at first. It becomes more a conscious, deliberate process in the teen and adult years. The child learns techniques, procedures, and mental tricks that help him make up for his weaknesses.

For instance, the child who has a terrible time with organizing tasks learns to make and follow lists—from morning to night. The one with sequencing problems learns to outline his total day. The child with poor spelling carries a dictionary to every college class. The one with writing problems learns to type or use the word processor. The impulsive child learns to count to ten before reacting.

Through the combination of physical maturation and learning, most children with ADHD do compensate, at least partially, for their dysfunctions and move on to varying levels of success as they approach the teen and adult years.

No, children do not "outgrow" ADHD. But they do overcome it.

There Is a Catch

There is one catch in this scenario of progressive improvement, however. Without proper management, the child with ADHD finds himself in constant conflict with his environment. His inefficiency in learning, general disorganization, and disruptive behavior result in failure to meet the expectations of his parents, teachers, and peers. The relationship between the child, his parents, and his teachers is often strained. There are few opportunities for reward and praise. after receiving predominantly negative feedback, he becomes progressively more aware of not pleasing important people in his life. This leads to loss of self-confidence and self-acceptance, which, in turn, leads to anxiety and frustration. Since he is not getting many positive strokes in his daily life, he is likely to adopt acting-out and attention-getting behaviors—showing off, arguing, deliberate disobedience—in a vain attempt to get the attention and recognition he so dearly wants. But this type of behavior only leads to more conflict and frustration.

The child whose ADHD is unrecognized and untreated is at high risk of developing an intense sense of failure and inadequacy, leading to low self-esteem. Thus emotional adjustment problems arise about the time the original neurological dysfunctions are resolving. In the long run, these secondary emotional adjustment disorders are more limiting and crippling than the original neurological impairments. A new cycle of failure and identity confusion can result.

Therefore, early recognition and management is of absolute urgency. Proper management will prevent, or lessen, the development of these secondary emotional adjustment disorders. Proper management also aids the child in building on his strengths in order to overcome his weaknesses.

The Plague of Parental Guilt

We were about halfway through our conference when Danny's mother paused. She blurted out quickly, "I'm so glad you said that."

"What do you mean?" I asked, perplexed.

"What you said about attention defect disorder being a physical problem and not the parent's fault." She paused again.

"Since Danny was a toddler, he has been very hard to control," she added. "I've been told by everyone—aunts, friends, teachers, perfect strangers—that if I would discipline him more, or if I would spend more time with him, or if I were a better parent, he wouldn't be so disruptive. I have felt like a total failure."

After a deep sigh, she whispered, "I felt so guilty."

As a parent and as a pediatrician, I know well this sense of guilt expressed so vividly by Danny's mom. Guilt must be the most common emotion shared by parents.

Parents can find all sorts of things, from small to gigantic, to feel guilty about. I see this every day in my office. Just last week, a mother brought her fifteen-year-old son, Jimmy, to see me. He had symptoms of a cough and congestion.

After my examination, I diagnosed Jimmy as having a common cold.

"Well," his mother replied, "I just knew I shouldn't have let him go on that hike in the rain. See, he got sick."

Jimmy's mother was reacting just like most parents. When something happens to a child, the parents automatically look inward to find some reason to take the blame. The brain searches its memory banks until it comes up with some event, often trivial, and the parent focuses on this as the cause of the problem. The child's problems, reasons the parent, sure are the result of something he or she has done or neglected to do. I see this kind of situation in my office every day. In fact, I spend much of my time helping parents understand that their child's minor and major ills are not their fault.

If You Were a Better Parent ...

This guilt may occur even when children are average, attractive, and well-adjusted. Parents then are beset with the idea that they could have done still better and could have inspired such children to be brilliant, beautiful, and perfectly adjusted. Popular magazines, psychological literature, and visual media often convey the message that whatever bothers children is directly related to what the parents did or did not do.

But the vulnerability to guilt is even truer for parents of boys and girls with ADHD and other learning disabilities. These parents have been told in words as well as in looks a thousand times, "Why can't you control that child?" Like Danny's mom, they have been confronted by well-intentioned friends and strangers with admonitions and advice. Implied behind all the advice and looks is the message, "If you were a better parent ..."

Concern

As a pediatrician, I am very concerned about such parental guilt. Few things are as destructive to healing as guilt. Guilt leads to negative, unproductive, and defensive actions by parents. Parents suffering under the burden of guilt are likely to deny that their child has a real problem. If they can deny the problem, they can deny their guilt in producing it.

When forced to admit that a problem exists, they are likely to become overprotective, caving into the child's whims, reluctant to take the hard steps necessary for healing and remediation. More importantly, guilt that is not dealt with honestly is likely to lead to parental stress or even depression. Such reactions then limit the parent's ability to cope energetically with the daily needs of family and child.

So ... we want to banish parental guilt by openly confronting it. Thus, for us to move on in helping ourselves manage the attention deficits and other learning disabilities, we must deal with this parental guilt.

Dealing with Guilt

The first step in dealing with this parental guilt is to learn the facts. Parents of children with attention deficit disorder and other developmental and/or learning disabilities need help in realizing that these are physical conditions, like diabetes. They are caused by multiple genetic and environmental influences.

ADHD, for example, is not a behavioral disorder that grows out of bad parenting; rather, its roots lie in the biological makeup of the person. ADHD children come equally from all kinds of families: poor and rich, strict and permissive, loving and distant. While certain techniques of discipline and parenting are a part of the treatment process, the lack of discipline or love does not cause ADHD.

A parent who is confused on this point should talk to a knowledgeable and understanding physician who can explain the details of the child's illness and its causes. Looking at the facts will help parents accept their lack of guilt intellectually. This step is usually necessary before emotional acceptance occurs.

If a parent feels that in some way he or she has inadvertently made mistakes in parenting, he or she needs to confront these feelings. This may involve talking about it with a competent counselor, pastor, or other compassionate listener. All parents need to accept the fact that no one is perfect. As parents, we will all make mistakes because we are human.

One of the best ways of dealing with guilt is to get involved with others. It helps to find other parents who are struggling with the same issues, either through formal organizations or casually. Becoming involved in community organizations that help children at risk is also a good antidote to the poison of guilt.

Along with these steps, parents can cope with their guilt by remaining whole persons even while caring for a child who demands more than ordinary attention and energy. Sacrificial tendencies, excessive attention to the child, or the neglect of all other aspects of living may take the mind off the problem temporarily, but they do not lead to productive or healthy living for parent or child. The child will be able to develop to his or her fullest potential when provided an atmosphere of confidence and calmness.

As parents who suffer from guilty feelings look outside of themselves, they can return from their self-imposed exile to a world of meaning and hope. Rather than nurse the guilty feelings, parents can move beyond them into something constructive. To parents, the message is, "God has accepted you and your child. Now accept yourself."

For Thought and Discussion

1. Chapter 4 lists the five basic steps in the management of the child with ADHD.

    A. Which of these steps have you taken already?

    B. Which ones will be hard for you?

    C. Which ones will be easy for you?

2. Which areas are you most concerned about right now?
    (Circle all the items you are concerned about. Then rate in order from one to five the ones you are most concerned about.)

> Behavior at school
> Behavior at home
> Behavior at play (peer relationships)
> Academic achievement
> Discipline
> Chores
> Homework
> Following directions

    (By listing the behaviors you are most concerned about, you will be better prepared to look for answers as you read this section. Also, by having written your concerns down, you will be more likely to ask about these when you talk to a professional who may be able to give you guidance.)

3. Have you been bothered by guilt regarding your child's condition? Why? What do you feel most guilty about? Why?

CHAPTER FIVE

Removing Aggravating Factors

ATTENTION deficit/hyperactivity disorder is a specific developmental condition with a defined set of characteristics. Although a varied spectrum of severity exists, children with ADHD demonstrate a consistent and typical pattern of behavior and neurological function.

However, this "pure" picture is often complicated by the presence of other developmental or emotional dysfunctions. Several "co-morbid" conditions are described by professionals working with ADHD children. Russell Barkley in his book, *Attention Deficit Hyperactivity Disorder, Diagnosis, and Treatment,*[2] states that co-morbidity "means that children with one disorder have a high likelihood of having a second." Several such conditions overlap with, and complicate, ADHD more often than would be expected by chance.

Common Co-Morbid Conditions

Let's look at some of the more common co-morbid conditions that may exist with ADHD:

Language-based learning disabilities. Central language processing disorders can mimic, and certainly complicate, the expression of attention disorders. For decades clinicians and educators have observed a significant overlap between children with ADHD and various language-

2   Barkley, Russell, *Attention Deficit Hyperactivity Disorder, Diagnosis, and Treatment.* New York: Guilford Press, 1990, 53.

based learning disabilities. As recently as two decades ago, professionals in the field tended to lump children with these related developmental disabilities together into the diagnostic category of minimal brain dysfunction. Attention, hyperactivity, and language-processing disorders were thought to be different ends of the continuum within this diagnosis. Recently the trend is to define the various diagnostic categories more precisely.

A recent study at the University of Georgia evaluated thirty children with central language processing disorder (CAPD). The incidence of ADHD in this group was found to exceed 50 percent, far greater than would be expected in the population at large (3–5 percent). While the authors suggested caution because of the overlap in symptoms between the two groups, this study strongly points to a link between the two. Certainly more studies with larger numbers of children are needed to define this association.

While many children with ADHD have no evidence of language-based learning disability, there are many children in which ADHD and a learning disability co-exist. I have seen children who have gone for years without treatment for their ADHD because all their academic problems were blamed on their language dysfunction. The attention problems and poor organization were thought to be secondary. On the other hand, I know of children who have not received serious evaluation of their reading and spelling underachievement because their poor grades were blamed on their attention deficit disorder. When a child has been diagnosed with either ADHD or language processing dysfunction, the child should be carefully observe for evidence of the other condition.

Oppositional Defiant Disorder. While children with ADHD may disobey and at times seems to resist discipline, they are not typically defiant. Their lack of compliance is most likely due to impulsiveness and failure to think before they act. They also have difficulty associating their behaviors with consequences. But they want to please and tend to be unhappy with their failure to live up to expectations.

Oppositional defiant disorder (ODD) is characterized by a pattern of negative, hostile, and defiant behavior. Children with this disorder easily lose their temper, purposely annoy others, openly defy authority, refuse to comply with rules, and argue often. They may be resentful, angry, spiteful, and vindictive. ODD is defined by a pattern of such behavior over a long period that is not due to temporary stresses or provocations. Oppositional defiant disorder is more common in males. Over time, ODD is likely to be associated with low self-esteem, low frustration tolerance, temper outbursts, poor peer relationships, and school underachievement.

Conduct Disorder. Children with conduct disorder exhibit a basic disregard for the rights of others and ignore age-appropriate norms of behavior. They may be cruel to other people and animals, fail to respect others rights (i.e., steal, misuse property), and ignore common rules of conduct. This pattern of behavior exists over a long period of time. It significantly disrupts the child's relationships and adjustments to common life situations, such as home and school.

Poor school performance, a greater frequency of school suspensions, and incidence of substance abuse are seen in children and adolescents with conduct disorders. These dysfunctional behaviors may begin in middle childhood but become more prominent in adolescence.

Tourette's Syndrome. Tourette's Syndrome (or Tourette's Disorder, as it is sometimes called today) is characterized by the onset during childhood of multiple tics of various kinds (both motor tics and vocal tics) that may fluctuate in severity. The currently accepted essential diagnostic criteria include onset before the age of twenty-one years, multiple involuntary motor tics, one or more vocal tics, the waxing and waning of the tics, the gradual replacement of old tics with new ones, the absence of other medical explanations for the tics, and the presence of tics for more than one year.

Along with the tics, there may be obsessive compulsive tendencies, excessive anxiety, sleep disorders, learning difficulties, and impulsive behaviors. A variety of behavior/emotional problems have been identified in children with Tourette's Syndrome. Whether these behavioral problems are related to tic severity, a direct consequence of having a stigmatizing condition, or an underlying part of the developmental condition is not clearly delineated.

ADHD has been reported to occur in 35 to 65 percent of children with Tourette's Syndrome. The treatment of children with attention deficit/hyperactivity disorder with co-morbid Tourette's Syndrome is controversial. The major confounding factor is that stimulant medications may provoke or intensify the tics. The stimulants do not cause the tics, but if a child is predisposed to tics, the use of the stimulants may hasten the expression of tics or aggravate them when they are present. While the stimulants may help the child with ADHD and Tourette's, they should be used with caution.

If behavior and educational approaches are not successful for the child with Tourette's and ADHD, then a trial with other types of medication should be considered.

Depression. It is well know that psychological depression is the most common emotional disorder affecting adults. The fact that depression is also very common in children and adolescents is less well known. Preteens and adolescents are particularly vulnerable to some degree of depression even under the best of circumstances. Children living with the stresses of ADHD are even more vulnerable. The frustration due to having to work harder to keep up academically, the constant negative feedback that is all too common, and the difficulty getting along with peers sets children up for depression. The usual low self-esteem experienced by many children with ADHD underlies their vulnerability.

A common sign suggestive of depression is a sudden drop in grades and performance in other activities, such as sports or music. Depressed children or adolescents will tend to be moody and easily frustrated. They seem sad and have more trouble enjoying things they have enjoyed in the past. They often will withdraw and be less able to cope socially.

Depression in children and adolescents is likely to be a reaction to circumstances and come on over a short period of time. Chronic, long-term depression is less common.

This reactive depression is probably the most common co-morbid condition seen in children with ADHD. Fortunately, depression is also the most effectively treated of all the co-morbid conditions. Recognition, counseling, and sometimes short-term antidepressant medication will usually overcome the depression fairly quickly.

Bipolar Disorder. Children with Bipolar Disorder tend to be moody, irritable, and often defiant. They may display varying degrees of inattention and impulsive tendencies that can be confused with the symptoms of ADHD. While such children are often bight, they may underachieve in school due to inconsistent performance. Children who are overly defiant and moody should be evaluated for Bipolar Disorder and/or depression prior to being diagnosed as ADHD.

Asperger's Syndrome. Asperger's Syndrome is a developmental disorder that affects a child's ability to relate to others and to socialize and communicate effectively. Children with Asperger's Syndrome tend to be socially awkward and exhibit an all-absorbing interest in certain topics. Asperger's Syndrome is considered to be one of the Autism Spectrum Disorders with a higher level of intellectual function. Children with Asperger's often show signs of ADHD, such as hyperactivity, short attention span, and impulsivity. The key difference is the social and relational problems that are always present with Asperger's Syndrome but not with ADHD alone. However, children with Asperger's may be helped considerably when the ADHD symptoms are treated effectively.

Confronting Co-Morbidity

Each of these conditions will affect the child's behavior and performance in specific ways. Many of the symptoms will mimic the functional disarrangements we see in ADHD. Certainly the presence of any one of these co-morbid conditions in association with ADHD will make life harder for the child, the parents, and other helpers.

Let us consider some practical implications of co-morbidity for those involved in caring for children with attention deficits and other behavior and learning conditions. The presence of a co-morbid condition, particularly oppositional defiant disorder or conduct disorder, definitely complicates the long-range progress of attention deficit disorder. The chance of long-term social and behavioral maladjustment is greatly increased in the presence of any of these co-morbid conditions.

It is important that any child who has learning or behavior problems has a complete evaluation in order to detect all potential areas of dysfunction. The presence of ADHD, as well as any co-morbid condition, should be uncovered as early as possible. Parents and professionals should remember that the presence of one dysfunction does not exclude the presence of another.

For example, many children with language-based learning disabilities have ADHD without hyperactivity that may not be recognized for several years. When the ADHD is not treated, the child will fail to maximize the educational interventions available to him. On the other hand, a child with obvious ADHD may be treated medically with some improvement but still struggle academically because the learning issues have not been fully identified and managed.

It is not always easy to find the skilled resources to deal will all of these complex issues, but they do exist. There are many excellent clinical psychologists, child psychiatrists, behavioral pediatricians, and other mental health professionals who are well-trained and experienced in clinical diagnosis.

Generally, parents should look for a mental health professional who specializes in children and who has expertise in behaviorally oriented approaches to treatment. To select a mental health practitioner, parents can ask a trusted health or school professional to make a referral. Parent groups often have the "inside scoop" on the local mental health resources and may provide helpful direction.

For the disruptive behavior disorders, such as oppositional defiant disorder and conduct disorder, some form of behavioral management and parent training will be a necessary part of the treatment strategy.

This may suggest to some that parents of such children are inadequate and at fault, but this is not the case. What it really means is that extraordinary management efforts are needed. This involves providing parents with behavioral management techniques and relationships so they can function as round-the-clock therapists for their child.

Effective parent training involves learning several specific techniques for modifying behavior, developing an effective plan for managing the child's behavior, putting the plan into effect, and revising and fine-tuning the plan to achieve the goals of better child behavior and parent-child relationships. At first this means a lot of work for parents. Very soon, though, parents find that they spend less time and energy managing their child's behavior, and family life becomes much more pleasant.

It is important that a comprehensive management plan be outlined that focuses on the total child, including whatever co-morbid conditions may be present.

Summary

In addition to the use of medication and behavior modification for inattention and impulsive behavior, intensive behavioral and psychiatric care may be necessary for oppositional or conduct disorders or specialized medical management needed for Tourette's syndrome. Successful outcomes are attainable with the child who has ADHD and other co-morbid conditions, but success comes with a great deal of hard work. Effective management requires close teamwork between parents, educators, physicians, and mental health specialists.

For Thought and Discussion

1. Do you think your child might have any of the co-morbid conditions discussed in this chapter? Which one(s)?

2. What behavioral symptoms suggest the presence of such a co-morbid condition?

3. What resources are available to help you evaluate your child's specific needs?

4. Have you discussed these concerns with your child's doctor or counselor?

CHAPTER SIX

Organization and Structure—Their Basic Need

Topsy-Turvy World

"I have tried everything, and nothing works," Mrs. Wilson told me at our first meeting as she reviewed her frustrations with Mark's behavior.

We can easily understand Mrs. Wilson's frustration, and those of all parents of children with ADHD, if we remember that the children, in varying degrees, lack appropriate control in the areas of attention, impulsiveness, and activity. Due to immaturity of brain organization, they simply cannot control, organize, and coordinate their actions as can other children their age.

Theirs is a topsy-turvy, upside-down world. They cannot "get it all together" and work consistently toward a goal without wandering off in all directions, both literally and figuratively. This disorganized approach to life is a function of their attention deficit, which makes it difficult for them to "stop, look, and listen." The result is frustration and failure for them in their daily relationships and customary pursuits in the home, classroom, and play with their peers.

The child's actual behavior is determined by the interrelationship between the underlying ADHD, individual personality traits, and the environment. These three factors interact with each other to produce the observed behavior of the child. For example, a child with very mild hyperactivity may not be a behavior problem in a calm, well-controlled, low-key family.

A child with a mild attention deficit may perform well in a small, organized classroom but bomb royally in a loud, distractible classroom. An overly impulsive child may be a total disaster in an inconsistent family but be at least partially manageable in a well-disciplined family. However, in the best of family and school environments, the child with moderate to severe ADHD will have significant problems in relationships as well as in performing ordinary, expected tasks.

Additional methods of management must be employed to have optimal performance and a healthy long-term outcome.

As mentioned earlier, successful management involves a combination of methods carried out over time. Becoming informed about the developmental nature of attention deficit is the first step. The next important step is the provision of a *cocoon of structure, organization, and consistency.* That's what this chapter is about.

The Structured, Supportive Environmental Cocoon

Since children with ADHD cannot effectively organize themselves, they function best in a world that is itself structured and organized. Their physical and psychological environment needs to be structured and consistent. This involves several components, which we will discuss in detail:

- Structure of time and place
- Effective, attention-holding communication
- Anticipation and avoidance of pressure points
- Effective discipline (proper use of behavioral techniques)
- Support of self-esteem
- Attention to specific problem behaviors, such as impulsiveness, hyperactivity, and learning disorders

Structure of Time and Place

Most children as well as adults, when left on their own, eventually will fit their daily routine into some sort of pattern that allows them to function successfully. Due to their internal disorganization, however, children with ADHD fail to do this effectively. They have difficulty focusing on a goal and aiming at it. Their increased susceptibility to distractions makes it difficult for them to stay focused on what is important at any given time.

The more unstructured, disorganized, and distracting the environment, the more the child is disorganized and disoriented as to his goals. This, in turn, leads to confusion and frustration, which leads to more disorganized, unsuccessful behavior. Thus in an unstructured, unregulated environment, the child is caught up in a spiraling web of deteriorating behavior. The more inconsistent and unpredictable the environment, the more disorganized the child's behavior becomes. This then induces more disorganization and inconsistency in his environment. The downward spiral of confusion and frustration goes on and on … and on.

An environment that calms, organizes, and structures the child's life is one of the primary steps in a strategy for success. The following techniques are basic.

1. *The first step is to provide a dependable time structure to the child's day.*

This means providing a predictable, dependable daily routine. Some elements of this are:

- Getting up the same time every day
- Regular daily schedule
- Regular routine for school, play naps, etc.
- Regular time for homework
- Regular bedtime

Such a regular, dependable routine does several things for the child. Each planned activity presents him a framework on which he can hang his day. The set routine gives him short-term goals to work toward. The time structure acts like handrails on the stairs that help the child keep his behavior more goal directed. Having certain activities to do at specific times makes him less likely to wander off into distracting, bothersome behavior.

In implementing such a time structure, the parent first decides on what would be a desirable daily pattern that fits the parents', as well as the child's, needs. At this point, it would be helpful to sketch out the daily schedule. The parents need to make sure the key elements (getting up, meals, school, bedtime) are such that they can enforce them consistently. They then discuss the schedule with the child.

The parents do not have to make a big production out of this scheduling task. They might simply say something like this: "This is going to be our schedule. Let's discuss it." If the child is old enough, the schedule can be written and posted in his room or some other conspicuous place. An older child (seven or eight or older) might participate in determining the contents of the schedule. Once the schedule has been determined, the parent enforces it consistently but gently.

This does not mean that the family must live a totally monotonous, unchanging life for the sake of this one child. But the day-to-day routine of the child should be as consistent as possible within the family's power to make it so. Certainly, there will be times when a break in the routine is needed. When change in this regular routine is necessary, however, it helps to prepare the child ahead of time and clearly state what you expect of him or her.

2. *The next step is the structure of place.*

"A place for everything and everything in its place" is more than a motto for the person with ADHD. It is a necessity. A search for a lost baseball glove can be a frustrating experience for a normal ten-year-old. But for a ten-year-old with ADHD, it can be a disaster, ending in an emotional explosion. Such problems can be prevented by helping the child organize his world (at least his room and his belongings) so there is a place for everything.

This could involve other elements, such as:

- A regular, non-distracting place to do homework.
- Labels on drawers and shelves to help the child locate the contents. (Some parents have successfully used color codes on drawers and shelves.)

- In strange new surroundings, such as on vacation, at a new school, or when visiting friends, it helps to take the child on a tour and show him the layout and locations of important particulars of the area.

An Ounce of Prevention

"An ounce of prevention is worth a pound of cure" is an old saying with a lot of experience to back it up. In no situation is this truer than in dealing with the behavior of the child with ADHD. It is much easier, and much less nerve-racking, to head off frustration and explosive situations than it is to soothe frayed nerves and mend ruptured plans after the explosion.

Some proven preventative measures are:

1. *Avoid problem situations when you can.*
2. Some potentially difficult situations and tips for dealing with them are:

    - Adult-oriented activities, such as parties, receptions, and recitals, particularly those of long duration.
    - Activities involving large groups of people.
    - Of course, you cannot always avoid these activities. But when you can, you probably will be better off doing so. At the right, time you may then introduce your child to these difficult events and activities in small doses.
    - Get a sitter when you can. Mom and Dad need a chance to enjoy adult activities without having to corral an active child. Parents should not feel guilty about using a sitter. In fact, this can be one of the most important coping mechanisms. The parents need a break from the active child, and the child needs a break from the parents.
    - If the whole family needs to attend a social event that will be difficult for the child, make the visit as short as possible with provisions for leaving when and if the child reaches his limits.

- Prepare the child ahead of time for a change in the schedule, and inform him of what to expect.
- Bring along a series of relatively quiet games, books, or other activities of interest to the child.

2. *Plan ahead when you can.*

Sometimes you cannot avoid the frustrating situations. You have no other option but to take the child to the store, to the cafeteria, or on a visit with your friends. When such potentially explosive changes in the routine must occur, prepare your child for them. Tell him well in advance what will happen and what you expect of him. If possible, plan short, interesting activities that will help occupy his time. While shopping, involve the child directly by having him read the shopping list or push the cart. One parent found a creative way to maintain control of the child in restaurants by playing tic-tac-toe on the napkins or other paper while waiting for the meal. Positive interaction with the child often heads off many negative conflicts.

3. *Avoid overstimulation when possible.*

Ideally, the child should have his own room. This may not always be possible; if not, a screened area in a shared room would be helpful. He can apply himself more constructively if he has a quiet place, free of distractions, in which to work. You may notice that your hyperactive child really goes wild at exciting events, such as special outings (circuses, movies, picnics) and holidays. Do not let the stimulation get out of hand if you can help it. It helps to prepare the child in advance for what will happen and what behavior you expect.

Get Their Attention

Due to his short attention span and poor short-term memory, the child with ADHD typically has difficulty carrying out instructions that are simple for others. For example, the normal child might be able to follow these directions: "Go undress, take a bath, brush your teeth, and get ready for bed."

But to the child with ADHD, such fairly simple instructions are confusing. He may get his clothes off only, to become distracted and begin to play. The parent, finding him dawdling, becomes angry.

A more appropriate way of handling this situation is to give short, concise instructions one at a time: "Please get undressed now, Jimmy."

When the child is undressed, say, "Now it is time to take your bath."

Once they have done this, other instructions can be given one at a time.

The same applies to chores: Rather than say, "Go clean up the yard," it is better to say, "Go rake the leaves." When this is done say, "Pick up the paper," etc.

Continue giving step-wise instructions until the job is completed. (This technique can also be applied very successfully to schoolwork.)

Remember, make the directions short, concise, and to the point.

There will come a time when you will say, "Jimmy, go undress," and when you check on him, he will have undressed, taken his bath, brushed his teeth, and climbed into bed reading a book. But this does not happen all at once. It comes after a long pattern of deliberately structuring and organizing the environment for him.

When you must have the child's undivided attention, you will need to override the extraneous stimuli competing with you.

A couple of practical maneuvers will help this:

1. *Use Touch.*

Gently put your arm around the child or your hand on his shoulder and then speak, giving him instructions, directions, praise, or criticism. Physical contact will overpower most other competing distractions and help the child more efficiently focus on you. (And, as a result, understand and remember what you have to say.)

2. *Use eye contact.*

With a soft but firm voice, ask the child to come to you and look in your eyes. Then speak. Such eye contact has vast potential as a communication tool and will, like physical touch, tend to override external competing distractions.

Consistent Discipline

This is a most important component of the supportive environmental cocoon. In fact, we devote a whole chapter to a discussion of the useful techniques of discipline (chapter 8). It is very important that the parents' rules and expectations for the child be clear, firm, and consistent. They should be clear in the sense that the parent communicates definitely to the child what is expected of him and what the consequences of his behavior will be. They should be firm in the sense that the parent sticks by the rules he or she sets. They should be consistent in that the rules are the same day in and day out, from parent to parent and place to place.

Who Is the Leader?

Often as I work with families with ADHD children, I find that other family members unknowingly conform themselves to the disorganization and confusion of the child rather than adapting the child to a consistent family environment. This occurs as the family tries one form of management after another for short periods of time. Seeing no immediate results, they then try something else. The harder they try, the more disordered their efforts become. The family routine follows the erratic patterns of the child rather than the child adjusting to the family. When the situation reaches such an impasse, it may take drastic reordering of the family routine to return to a stable and more normal course, but the effort is well worth it.

The Overriding Goal

The goal is to provide an absolutely predictable environment. Rather than being cruel, this is a caring thing to do—the result is a happier and more productive child who can cope better with his day-to-day challenges. Failure to provide some degree of structure will likely result in an unhappy, frustrated child with stunted emotional growth. The child may protest when he is reminded to put his baseball glove back on the top shelf of the closet, but he will be rewarded the next time he goes to get it. The main purpose of regimentation is therapeutic.

Remember, the child with ADHD lacks internal organization. As he lives in an externally organized and consistent environment, he eventually builds into his own system some of this external organization and consistency. There will come a time when he is more and more capable of internal control and is able to plan ahead, stop, look and listen, and function productively on his own. For some, their day of success seems slow in coming, but it will come. It will come sooner if the child is provided with a structured, organized pattern to follow.

Looking for the Positive

The child with ADHD is persistently engaging parents and teachers with his disruptive impulsive, overactive behavior. Adults find it necessary to intervene often, control, redirect, admonish, and stand between the child and disaster!

It is easy for adults in such circumstances to find themselves primarily focusing on the negative side of the child's behavior and character. The child's positive traits are overshadowed by the high profile of his bothersome behavior. Adults then fall into a pattern of only interacting with the child in negative, corrective, limit-setting ways.

However, if those of us working with the child take time to reflect, we can see that the ADHD child does have his or her own repertoire of likeable, positive qualities. It is absolutely necessary to deliberately look for these desirable qualities if we really want to help the child "grow through" his ADHD to become a self-actualizing, self-disciplining adult.

Sleep and ADHD

The questionnaire parents complete in our office to provide medical history and developmental background asks several questions regarding sleep:

Does your child have difficulty falling asleep?

Does he or she awaken frequently during the night?
Does he or she have difficulty awakening in the morning?
Does he or she have restless sleep?

In this non-statistical survey of parental observations, more than 70 percent of the parents reported that their child with ADHD has some type of problem with sleep. As in our informal poll, sleep disturbance is commonly perceived to be associated with attention deficits. However, objective confirmation has been sketchy. Now in the last few years, researchers have given some attention to this issue.

Barbara Trommer, MD, and associates[3] studied sleep disturbance in children with attention deficit disorder. The researchers compared ADHD children who were not taking medication at the time with matched controls. Fifty-three percent of the ADHD children took longer than thirty minutes to fall asleep, while only 23 percent of the controls experienced such delay. Fifty-five percent of the ADHD children were described as being tired on awakening, while only 27 percent of the control children did. The ADHD children also awakened more frequently during the night than the controls.

Bonnie Kaplan, PhD, and associates[4] also sought to use objective means to study the sleep of children with ADHD. In addition to questionnaires, they had parents monitor their child's sleep over time and keep a log of their observations. They found that ADHD children did have more nighttime wakening than control children. Children with ADHD in their study got up at night twice as often as the control children. They also found that ADHD children took fewer, and shorter, naps during the day.

Thus objective evidence confirms the longstanding subjective impressions that children with ADHD do have significant sleep disturbances.

How Much Sleep

While data is sparse on the average hours of sleep needed by ADHD children, clinical observations suggest that most fall at either end of the

---

3   Trommer, B, *Annals of Neurology*, 24:2, p. 322.
4   Kaplan, B, *Pediatrics* 80:6, 839.

spectrum. Many have short sleep requirements. From infancy, they need only minimal sleep. These children may also have trouble going to sleep, and they wake up early. On the other hand, some ADHD children seem to have increased sleep needs. They fall asleep immediately and are slow getting up in the morning. It is as if they need much more time to recharge their exhausted batteries

Causes of Sleep Disturbances

The reasons for children with attention deficit disorder having more frequent sleep disturbances are not entirely clear.

Sleep is an autonomic phenomenon reflecting cyclic changes in arousal. Previous studies have documented changes in sleep patterns in various conditions, such as depression, characterized by alterations in central nervous system arousal. Since faulty arousal mechanisms have been implicated as an underlying problem in attention deficit disorder, the presence of sleep disturbances in children with ADHD is not surprising.

Barbara Trommer in her article suggests the possibility of "cognitive hyperactivity." This is described as the "inability to stop thinking." The ADHD child simply cannot turn off cognitive activity in order to let the brain relax.

The ADHD child's difficulty in regulating physiologic cycles, such as the circadian (day/night) rhythm, plays a part. The child with attention deficit may be vulnerable to what is called "delayed sleep phase," wherein the child can achieve a normal amount of sleep, but the sleep begins and ends later by an hour or two. Such a child falls asleep at the same hour, night after night, regardless of bedtime or parental demands. A family may put their child to bed, for example, at 7:00 p.m., only to be confronted by three hours of struggles, fights, excuses, requests, and demands. No matter what the parents do, the child falls asleep at a very late hour. The exact hour of sleep seems to coincide with the child's physiological readiness for sleep.

In fact, as in non-ADHD children with sleep problems, many factors likely interact to produce the frequent sleep disturbances in children with ADHD.

More recently, a variety of studies reported in the pediatric research literature have identified obstructive sleep apnea as a contributing factor of ADHD symptoms in certain children. In this condition, sleep is continually interrupted through the night due to blocking of air flow in the nose and throat. This condition is frequently caused by enlargement of the tonsils and/or the adenoids and nasal allergies. Obstructive sleep apnea should be suspected in any child with frequent or regular snoring or noisy breathing during sleep.

Significance

Regardless of the cause, the sleep problems in the child with ADHD are a significant disruption in his life and disturbs the family's accommodation to his developmental disorder. The parents become frustrated and then angry. They tend to see the sleep disruption as willful disobedience on the part of the child. They react, in turn, with threats, negative feedback, and verbal combat. This heightens tensions in the family, creates anger in the child, and results in even more delay in acquiring normal sleep. I often see families in which the conflict over sleep has become a major focus of distorted parent-child relationships.

When the delayed onset of sleep, or frequent awaking during the night, reduces the child's total sleep, the child is not likely to cope as well with the demands of his attention deficits and impulsiveness. Lack of sleep may increase restlessness and hyperactivity during the day. A tired child has less endurance for work and is less likely to sustain effort in class or other endeavors.

Certainly sleep problems can play a significant role on many levels in the life of a child with attention deficit disorder and his family.

How to Help

The disrupted sleep of ADHD originates in the neurological dysrhythmia of the child's central nervous system. It may not be possible to completely alleviate the sleep problems with behavioral and environmental means. However, there are things that can be done to facilitate rest, decrease conflict, and make the situation more acceptable to all concerned.

Some suggestions:

1. *Establish regular, consistent routines and rituals surrounding bedtime and awakening.* Going to bed and getting up should be consistent from day to day. It is important to establish pleasant, rewarding routines about bedtime. Pleasant interaction between parent and child in which the child and the family relationships are affirmed should be the goal. Have a routine: take a bath, read a story, plan the next morning (set out clothes, etc.), say prayers, say good-night, go to sleep. Depending on the age of the child, parents can be involved in this process at varying levels of intensity.

2. *Parents need to remember that children with ADHD have a difficult time sequencing activities.* The parents may need to help the child structure the bedtime routine: "It's time for bed. Take off your clothes." Once this is done, the parent says, "Take your bath." Then the parent says something to the effect, "That's good. Now put on your pajamas and let's read our story."

Once "good-night" is said, the parent refrains from verbally interacting with the child. The parent should not threaten, scold, or argue. If the child gets out of bed or comes out of his room, the parent gently, but firmly, takes him back to his room and says, "It is bedtime. You are not allowed to be up."

3. *Parents must realize that the ADHD child may be physically unable to fall asleep right away.* It is appropriate to let the child read himself to sleep, listen to music, or use some other procedure that helps him to relax. As long as the child stays in bed, parents can be satisfied. The immediate goal is not to get the child to go to sleep on the parents' timetable but for him to learn to control himself and not be a disruptive influence to the rest of the family.

4. *Have a regular time of getting up in the morning.* This should be early enough that the child is not rushed or pushed in getting ready. Many ADHD children need time to "get the motor started" in the morning. It is best to let the child have his own alarm clock and wake up on his own. The child may need a checklist to go by in getting dressed in the morning.

If the child consistently goes to sleep late and has a difficult time getting up in the morning, he may be experiencing "delayed sleep phase." One method of treating this is to wake the child up earlier in the morning at a set time while sticking with a consistent, earlier bedtime.

5. *Enforce the expected sleep routine.* A child who awakens at night and comes to the parents' room should be gently but firmly taken back to his own bed. Simply say something like, "I'm sorry you are having trouble sleeping, but you must sleep in your own room."

Do not let the child start sleeping in your room. If you do so, you will have a very hard time changing this habit later.

6. *If your child has a major problem with falling asleep at night, or if he wakes frequently at night, talk with the child's physician.* Such a child may have a more severe disturbance in the rhythm of sleep. Medication may be used to help correct the neurological dysfunctions affecting sleep. The ADHD child is not usually helped by sedatives, however. In fact, he is likely to be overly stimulated by them. There are other medications, however, that may help normalize sleep.

There is increasing evidence that breathing problems during sleep due to upper airway obstruction may worsen the symptoms of ADHD. Such breathing problems can be due to large tonsils and/or allergies. If the child with ADHD snores excessively or seems to wake up frequently during the night, an evaluation by the physician for sleep apnea should be considered.

For Thought and Discussion

A: Establishing a regular schedule:

1. How consistent is your child's daily schedule now? (Rate on a scale of one to ten.)

Irregular and confused Organized and structured

1 2 3 4 5 6 7 8 9 10

2. What are some factors in your family that make consistent structure of time and place difficult?

3. What are some things about your family that may help you provide a more organized environment for your child?

4. Sketch out below a schedule you and your child can live with. Include such things as getting up, having breakfast, dressing, school or play, homework, chores, dinner, free time, bath, and bed.

(You may wish to write this schedule on a sheet of paper or a poster board and put it in your child's room or other prominent place to help all of you keep on track.)

B. Improving organizational skills:

1. Some problems your child has with organization:

2. Some ways you can help him/her become more organized and structured:

3. Some methods you can use to make sure your child hears what you say (i.e., gets the instructions straight):

C. Discovering your child's positive traits and behaviors:

1. Five things I like about my child's personality:

2. Five skills my child performs well:

3. Five desirable, helpful, or pleasant things my child did in the last week:

Now be honest. Ask yourself, "How many times have I acknowledged or complimented my child on these positive qualities?" Circle the number in the above list where you have made any kind of recognition of the child for his positive actions.

Everyone has some gift. Everyone has positive points. Let's look for these in our children.

Catch them being good, and tell them about it.

CHAPTER SEVEN

Medical Treatment

How It All Began

IN the early 1930s, Dr. Charles Bradley and his associates faced a difficult medical problem. Numerous adults and children with neurological impairment following a variety of illnesses suffered from seizures, headaches, and other symptoms, as well as behavior and learning problems. In those days, few medications were available to treat these neurological conditions. In desperation, Dr. Bradley attempted to treat the patients with what was even then an older class of drugs, the amphetamines.

During this study, Dr. Bradley observed an intriguing phenomenon. The patients' seizures and headaches did not get much better, but many of the hyperactive, distractible children and adults who had been so hard to manage reacted in an unusual way. Ordinarily these drugs function as stimulants—that is, in most people they increase activity and restlessness. But in these patients, they produced the opposite effect. These hyperactive and distractible patients were calmer, more cooperative, and able to learn more proficiently.

Since Dr. Bradley's pioneering discovery, numerous other researchers have shown the effectiveness of stimulant medication in helping children with hyperactivity and attention problems due to neurological dysfunction. This accidental discovery decades ago was a breakthrough in treatment.

By the 1940s and 1950s, the usefulness of the stimulants in treating hyperactivity and impulsivity was becoming well known. In the 1950s, newer forms of stimulants became available that were better tolerated than the older forms. This made treatment more practical.

The syndrome we now know as ADHD grew out of Dr. Bradley's discovery. Through decades of research and debate, medical treatment with stimulants has remained an integral part of the management of ADHD. Thanks to our increasing knowledge of brain physiology and chemistry, medical treatment is better understood and practiced today.

Since this initial discovery, a large store of information has accumulated regarding the medical treatment of the neuro-developmental condition we now call attention deficit disorder. In this chapter, we will explore the many ramifications of such medical treatment.

Concerns about Medical Treatment

Parents are often reluctant to "give drugs" for what appears to be a problem of behavior. This concern is understandable. Thus it is important to look rationally at this issue, considering the benefits against any possible risks.

The aim of medical treatment is not to "drug" the child into submission or to just get rid of obnoxious behavior. Rather, medical treatment is used to stimulate more normal functioning of those components of the neurological system that are not working up to their normal level. Indeed, the physical underpinnings of attention deficits, as developed in the recent medical literature, documents that there is an imbalance in the neuro-transmitter substances in the brain of people with ADHD. Thee neuro-transmitters are responsible for nerve impulse conduction in the control centers of the brain. Medication, properly used, helps "normalize" the levels of neuro-transmitters, allowing a healthier neurological functioning.

Choices

Stimulants have a long track record of effectiveness in the treatment of ADHD and related disorders. They have been used over many years and proven to be effective with a minimal of side-effects with the majority of children. However, for various reasons some individuals cannot tolerate the stimulants or they do not work well for others. Over the years, many different types of medicines have been evaluated for the treatment of ADHD. While other classes of drugs helped somewhat in some children, none have been as universally effective as the stimulants. The search for alternative forms of medical treatment continues, and exciting things are happening in pharmaceutical research. Some promising medications are on the horizon.

The following discussion refers to treatment with stimulants, which continues to be the mainstay of medical management.

Stimulants come in a variety of forms with varying dose sizes and length of duration. Common forms are as follows, with brand name and generic name:

Commonly Used Stimulants

Brand Name—Generic Name

Ritalin—methylphenidate

Concerta—extended release methylphenidate

Focalin—newer form of methylphenidate

Adderall—mixed amphetamine salts

Dexedrine—dextroamphetamine

Vyvanse—a unique relative of methylphenidate

What to Expect from Medication

Stimulants work by increasing the child's overall control of his or her disorganized activity, attention, and impulsiveness. A child responding positively to the medication is noted to be better organized, attentive, less impulsive, and more capable of self-monitoring. He *stops, looks, and listens* in a more appropriate way. Parents often note, with some relief, that the child is more compliant with discipline. The quality of school work tends to improve, not because the child is suddenly smarter, but because he is more efficient and less careless in his work. There is less emotional up and down.

The most widely accepted theory of how this happens is that the medication affects the chemical milieu of the brain, restoring a normal balance to this system. It is as if the medication *stimulates* the underfunctioning control center of the brain so it functions in a more normal manner. Thus, the brain is able to modulate and organize its output appropriately.

I must emphasize that the purpose of stimulant medication is not to tranquilize, dull, or control the child. Nor is the medication used to change the child's personality. Rather, the purpose is to restore the child's function to normal so he or she can control and organize his or her own behavior in a way appropriate to his or her age and personality.

What Are the Side Effects?

Certainly any medication has potential side effects. Potential benefits should always be weighed against any potential ill effects when any medication is prescribed. Stimulants have been used for years and have a good safety record. While they do have side effects, these are usually easily spotted. Such side effects are not likely to be serious at recommended doses and usually can be controlled by adjusting the way the medications are taken.

Potential side effects of stimulants can be summarized as follows.

Appetite suppression. Many children will have a mild decrease in the appetite when first starting on stimulants. The appetite typically returns to normal in a week or two. A few children will have a more persistent loss of appetite even at recommended doses. However, the degree of appetite loss can usually be controlled by regulating the amount and timing of the dose. A rare child will have more severe appetite suppression, resulting in weight loss. When this happens, change in dose and timing should be tried. If severe appetite loss persists, the medication will need to be discontinued. Taking the medication with or right after meals lessens the chance of appetite disturbance.

Sleeplessness. Due to an overactive stimulant effect, the stimulants can cause difficulty falling asleep for some children. Most children taking stimulants at regular doses during the day will not experience any problem with sleep. When sleep problems do occur, they are usually corrected by adjusting the amount and timing of the medication dose.

Rarely, sleep problems will be severe enough to require the discontinuing of medication. (However, it is important to realize that many ADHD children have a significant sleep disturbance as a part of their neurological dysfunction. Thus the medication may not be the cause of disrupted sleep.)

Decreased growth. Several years ago, reports in the medical literature suggested that stimulants might cause a decrease in the rate of growth in children. This concern has been studied extensively over the years. In fact, most children taking stimulants experience no problem with growth. A few children will have a fall off in their growth curve while on medication. However, when this occurs, it is related to the decreased appetite sometimes seen.

This should never be a problem in a child who is properly monitored. All children taking stimulants should have their height and weight measured and plotted on a growth curve regularly. If there is any evidence in loss of appetite or fall off in the growth pattern, the amount or timing of the medication can be altered to minimize effect on the appetite.

It also helps to provide periodic "medication holidays," such as on weekends and the summer, to minimize any effect on appetite.

Presence of movement disorders. As discussed in an earlier chapter, the child taking stimulants should be observed for any form of repetitive motor movement or tic. Eye blinking, head jerking, or mouth movements are example of such tics. Most medical experts do not believe that the stimulants actually cause the tics. However, in a person who is genetically susceptible, stimulants may precipitate the expression of the tic. Such occurrences should be reported to the supervising physician. (See chapter 4.)

Cardiovascular effects. Stimulants, like their relative caffeine, may cause some increase in the pulse rate and blood pressure at higher doses. At regular doses, these effects are minimal and appear to have no significant effects on the body. At higher than regular doses, such rapid heart rate (tachycardia) or arrhythmia (irregular heartbeats) may become more noticeable. Any evidence of irregular or rapid heartbeat should be reported to the physician. However, clinical studies have not shown any significant problem with arrhythmia or tachycardia in children taking recommended therapeutic doses. It is important to notify the physician of any family history of heart disease of any kind. If there a family history of heart disease, it is advisable to get an EKG prior to starting stimulant medication.

All of these side effects are uncommon at the recommended doses. When they do occur, they disappear quickly once medication is discontinued.

Toxic Reactions

Toxic reactions generally refer to the effect of the drug on the body when taken at higher than recommended doses or when the person is unusually sensitive to the physiologic effects. Such toxic reactions of stimulants are:

- Headaches, dizziness
- Severe loss of appetite with weight loss
- Agitation and irritability
- Severe sleeplessness
- Very rapid or irregular pulse
- Hallucinations—seeing, hearing and feeling things that are not there.

The occurrence of any of these symptoms should be reported to the physician immediately.

Schedules and Doses

Doses and schedules must be individualized and depend both on the characteristics of the specific medication being given as well as the unique response of each individual.

Until recently there were only a few ways the stimulants could be given. Primarily, a short-acting form of methylphenidate (Ritalin) and dextroamphetamine (Adderall, Dexedrine) were available. With these short-acting forms of the medication, two or three doses during the day are often required for optimal response. For the child who is having problems only at school, a morning dose alone may be sufficient. The more hyperactive child will likely need a dose in the morning, a dose at noon, and possibly another in the afternoon. As a dose wears off, the child reverts back to the hyperactive behavior, and this fluctuation confuses the child, as well as those people around him. Attention to the spacing of the doses is necessary to minimize this rebound.

More recently, long-acting forms of both methylphenidate and dextroamphetamine and their derivatives have been developed. With these the span of action can be as long as six to ten, even twelve, hours. These are particularly useful for the older child in middle and high school for whom taking multiple doses during the day is inconvenient and socially disconcerting.

Whether the child should take the medication on weekends or during the summer depends on various factors, such as the child's level of dysfunction and the kind of demands made on his coping resources. What is best for one child may not be best for another. Such decisions should be worked out in a cooperative effort by parents and physician.

When possible, the child should be given a periodic holiday from the medication. Some children do well without the medication for the summer. Others may skip just one or two weeks during the summer. Others may take holidays on weekends. For some children, any time off the medication is a disaster, and such holidays are not practical until they are older and more controlled.

When to Stop the Medication

The immediate, transparent answer would be, "When the child no longer needs it." But how do you make such a decision? In general this determination is made by observing the child's behavior and performance on and off the medication. Input from parents, teachers, and other observers is helpful. No actual test of any kind currently exists that gives a concrete answer to this question.

Some children grow out of their need for the medication after a year or two. Others will need it for several years. Overall, about one-third of the children can do well without the medication by the beginning of puberty (beginning of middle school). Another third can do well without it by the end of puberty (end of middle school). Another one-third will continue to benefit from medical treatment well into the teens or adulthood.

"I Did It Myself"

How does the taking of medication for attention deficits affect the child's view of himself or herself? Does the child become psychologically dependant on the drug? Does he see the medicine as a "good pill" he cannot function well without it? Such questions have often been asked by both parents and professionals.

A study, published in the *Journal of Consulting and Clinical Psychiatry* (Vol. 60, No. 2, 282–292) evaluated how children perceive themselves and their behaviors when taking medication for attention deficit disorder. Serial studies of twenty-eight boys with ADHD attending an eight-week summer day-camp program were undertaken. The boys were treated with methylphenidate (Ritalin) in standard doses or given a placebo. They were then asked to evaluate their own behavior. They were asked if various behaviors were caused by the medication, the influence of counselors, or their own effort.

The boys whose behavior improved with medication attributed their positive performance to their own effort and not to the medication. They attributed their negative, or unpopular, behavior to counselors or the medication.

Is this a reflection of real life or not? Apparently the stimulant medication did not change these children's natural humanity! When they were "good," they did it themselves; when they were "bad," it was the fault of someone else. How real!

The results of this study, however, do offer some additional reassurance that ADHD children are not likely to see medication as magic; and they seem to be less likely to become dependent on it. This parallels my experience, in which preteen children accept the medication in a matter-of-fact way. Teenagers, on the other hand, are more likely to resent having to take medication.

The Timing of the Dose of Medication

> My eight-year-old son is has been taking a short-acting medication for about a year for ADHD. It has made a tremendous difference in his grades at school. And, in general, his behavior is much better controlled. However, I notice a particular pattern: He is very hyper in the morning, but about thirty minutes after he takes his medication, he settles down and is much more controlled and attentive. However, by 10:30 or 11:00 a.m., his teacher notes that he becomes restless and the quality of his work falls off considerably. Is this a common pattern with Ritalin? Is there anything we can do to alleviate these peaks and valleys?

And here is another story:

> My six-year-old has been taking extended-released methylphenidate at breakfast for the past three months. He is doing wonderfully at school. His grades are now A's and B's. The teacher tells me he is well-behaved. But when he gets home in the afternoon, he is out of control. He is, if anything, more hyperactive than ever. And he is irritable, which is a definite change. What could be causing this? Would it help if he took a dose of Ritalin after school?

Both of these children are experiencing the effects of "medication rebound." One of the characteristics of stimulants, especially the short-acting ones, is the rapid adsorption into the body and rapid metabolism; its effect lasts about three to four hours. Once it is out of the system, the usual ADHD behaviors—hyperactivity, impulsiveness, and disorganization—return with a vengeance. Many children may become frustrated and irritable as they experience a resurgence of these driven behaviors.

In my experience, most children with significant hyperactivity and impulsiveness will perform better with one of the long-acting forms of medication. When rebound persists, a small dose of short-acting medication given after school will correct this rebound and allow the child to have a more normal afternoon. If needed, you should not hesitate to give this afternoon dose. From the perspective of the child's future, the relationships in the family are just as important as his achievement in school.

Potential problems with an afternoon dose are decreased appetite for dinner and difficulty falling asleep at bedtime. These problems can be minimized by adjusting the amount and timing of the medication.

In addition to giving multiple doses of medication, rebound may be managed by using one of the sustained-released forms of the medication. This will work for most children.

The various alternatives methods of medical treatment should be discussed frequently with the supervising physician. As parents and physician get to know the child's unique way of handling the stimulant medication, more effective adjustments can be made in the dosing schedule.

Vacation from Medication

> I have heard that it is a good idea for the child to take vacations from the medication. When should this be done? How is it done?

The *Physicians' Desk Reference* suggests that a person taking stimulants should have a break from the medication occasionally. There are several reasons why this is a good idea. If there is any appetite suppression with resultant decrease in weight gain or height growth, a vacation allows for catch-up growth. It also allows parents, physicians, and other observers to see how the child functions without the medication. Taking periodic holidays or vacations decreases the possibility that the child will have significant stimulant effects.

Some children do well taking the medication only on school days, thus having mini-vacations on weekends. Others can take all summer off, returning to the medication with the start of school. However, other children, particularly those who are more hyperactive and impulsive, may not be able to function well off the medication. In these children only small "vacations" of a day or two may be taken. As the child gets older and has more control over his ADD behavior, vacations can be more frequent and extensive.

There is no problem in starting and stopping the stimulants as needed. One does not have to be weaned off of them slowly.

Should the Child Take the Medication When He Is Sick?

> My child was recently ill with strep throat and home in bed. At the time, I was undecided about whether to give him his regular dose of Adderall. Should it be given when the child is sick?

Taking the medication when the child is acutely ill is optional. It the child is ill enough to stay home from school, or stay in bed, or if he or she is not eating well, then it would be best to suspend medical treatment temporarily. If, however, the child feels well enough to be up and about, or if he needs the control offered by the medication, he can continue to take it without a problem. If you have any question about a given situation, you should certainly talk with the child's physician.

My Child Is Not Hyperactive. Will Medication Help?

> My child has attention deficit disorder without hyperactivity. In fact, she is a likeable, easygoing child. But she has a very hard time focusing. Can medication help her?

Many people think that medication is given only to control behavior. They believe that if the child is not wildly active or terribly impulsive and causing havoc all around him, he is not a candidate for medication. However, this is a false impression.

In fact, some of the most dramatic successes with medical

treatment occur with children having attention deficit disorder without hyperactivity—who mainly have problems with attention, organization, and sequencing. With medication, function in school and in extra-curricular activities improves remarkably. Grades can go from failing to A's and B's in a short period of time. In fact, such children will often do well with quite modest amounts of stimulant medication.

Other Medicines

Stimulants have been the mainstay of drug treatment for attention deficit disorder and related syndromes for decades. Other drugs have come and gone, but none have proven as effective or safe as stimulants. However, they are not as effective for all children, and the search for other effective medicines continues. Recent studies suggest other drugs that are, to varying degrees, helpful for some children with ADD.

While not generally as effective as stimulants, certain anti-depressants can be helpful, particularly in those children for whom stimulants do not work and in children who have a major depressive component to their disorder. Anti-depressants are probably more useful in older teens and adults with ADD. Interestingly, these drugs also work on the dopamine pathways and target particularly the frontal lobe system.

Strattera is a non-stimulant that has been approved in recent years for the treatment of ADHD. While not as widely helpful as stimulants, Strattera is effective for some children and adults.

Other drugs are being studied and used clinically but have not been approved for use in children with ADD. Clonidine and its derivatives, used to treat high blood pressure in adults, is effective for some individuals with ADHD and tic disorders. A variety of other drugs help in certain situations, particularly in children with co-morbid conditions.

As we gradually learn more about brain chemistry in ADHD, the search for effective medication is more focused. Researchers are now looking at a variety of drugs that may be of value eventually.

Limitations of Medical Treatment

While dramatic turn-arounds can occur in the function of the ADHD child properly treated with medication, medical treatment is only one element is a comprehensive treatment plan. For optimal success, multiple strategies, such as wise use of discipline, behavior modification, educational planning, and family counseling, need to be a part of the management plan. Although medication is often necessary for other parts of the management plan to work, it is not a cure-all by itself.

The Need for Close Supervision

Any child taking stimulants needs to be monitored regularly by a physician. The child's progress should be evaluated and a check made for side effects. The child should be examined, his height, weight, and blood pressure measured, and any questions discussed.

Working as a Team

While the physician must ultimately manage the medical treatment program, he or she will of necessity rely on information from others in determining the diagnosis and monitoring the effectiveness of treatment. Important players in the medical treatment program in addition to the physician are the parents, teacher(s), and therapist if one is involved. The physician will depend on feedback, particularly from parents and teachers, in determining the relative effectiveness of the medical treatment program. This can be done through interviews as well as through the use of standardized questionnaires.

Other Forms of Treatment

While appropriate medication is central to the effective treatment of attention deficits, medical treatment is not the only therapy and needs to be used in cooperation with other helpful techniques. Some other proven methods of management are behavioral modification, academic accommodation, parent training, social skills training for the child, tutoring for specific learning disabilities, and individual counseling for the child and/or family. Families will likely need help in understanding and using these methods of treatment whether or not medical therapy is instituted.

The emphasis of this book is on a comprehensive management strategy that utilizes all of the available resources that have proven to be effective. The following chapters give practical guidance in the application of behavioral management and educational techniques.

For Discussion and Thought

1. How do you feel about medication for your child?

    a. Are you afraid of it? Why?

    b. Do you want to try medication? Why?

    c. What, or who, has influenced your ideas about medication the most?

2. Has your child tried medication before? If so what kind? What were the effects?

3. What are some questions you would like to ask the physician about medication if he or she recommended it?

4. How do you think your child would feel about medication?

SECTION THREE
STRATEGIES IN GROWING

CHAPTER EIGHT

Strategies in Discipline

A Common Concern

"I am very confused and frustrated about discipline," Mrs. Walters told me. "Arnold wants so badly to please; yet he's always breaking the rules and doing things he shouldn't. I know there are some things he cannot help, but I know he often can help what he does."

She paused to gather her thoughts. "And I don't know whether to be lenient or strict."

Mrs. Walters's confusion about discipline is shared by many other parents. This confusion, however, is not limited to parents of children with problems. Real confusion runs throughout society as to the goals of parenthood and how we can best attain them. Even when we know what we want our children to do, we often do not know how to get them to do it. To help clarify this confusion, we need to explore the meaning of discipline.

Special Discipline Needs

The typical symptoms of ADHD do, indeed, make discipline more difficult. The disordered activity, attention, and impulse control brings the child with ADHD into conflict with his environment much more frequently than other children. His attention problems often result in failure to complete tasks that have been assigned.

For example, when Sarah is told to take out the trash, she picks up the pail and starts out the door. Because she starts off running, she stumbles at the door and spills some of it. After recovering from this, she starts again. When she doesn't return with the pail in several minutes, her mom looks for her. Outside, the pail is sitting halfway to the trash bin and Sarah is off at the other side of the yard chasing a butterfly.

Sarah is not consciously disobeying. She, like so many with ADHD, has been led astray by her disorganized, wandering mind. Then, due to the *lack of impulse control*, she overreacts. As soon as she has acted, she thinks to herself, "Oops, I shouldn't have done that." But the deed is already done, and it usually gets her into trouble.

Lack of emotional control may lead the child to react in impulsive anger when rules are enforced. Again, he overreacts.

Then, too, children with *perceptual dysfunction* may not always understand the rules clearly. And of course, the poorly coordinated child is accident prone; he may be willing to dust the furniture but in the process may knock over two vases and a lamp.

Another common characteristic noted by parents is *difficulty profiting from experience (from trial and error)*. This frustrates the discipline process in that the child may need to be challenged over and over for the same infraction of the rules. Parents find themselves asking, "Will he ever learn?"

The actual methods of discipline used in these situations are essentially the same as those used with children in general. What is different is the extra dose of *patience, understanding, and consistency* with which the discipline is meted out.

Definition of Discipline

We often think of discipline only in negative terms. We equate it with punishment. The *New World Dictionary* defines discipline as "training to act in accordance to rules." It is derived from the Latin word meaning "to learn." Punishment is defined as "pain or penalty inflicted on a person for a crime or offense," and it is derived from the Latin word meaning "pain."

The real difference between discipline and punishment, however, is not so much in methods as in goals. Punishment seeks revenge and retribution; discipline seeks to produce right behavior and healthy feelings. Punishment attacks the child and his personality while discipline is aimed at the objectionable behavior.

Discipline seeks to impart to the child the right way to act and feel. Proper discipline says, "I love you, but I don't like what you did." When five-year-old Laura spills her juice on the table, punishment asks, "What does she deserve for this mess?" The answer may be scolding or spanking. Discipline asks, *"What can she learn from this?"* One thing she can learn, for example, is that people who make messes, either accidentally or on purpose, must clean them up.

Our Motives as Parents

The motives behind human behavior are as diverse as people. Some things we do in order to survive; some things we do out of a search for meaning and purpose in life. Some acts are motivated by individual needs. This is true of our discipline as well as other areas of human endeavor. Thus we should ask, *"Why am I disciplining as I am?"*

Sometimes we discipline our children because we are angry or frustrated; we are tired and our fuse is short. At other times, we may have a deep-seated need to be "the boss." In this case, discipline is an effort to establish the parents' authority or superiority over the child. Sometimes we discipline in order to make our children acceptable to other people—to keep them from embarrassing us.

All of us as parents are motivated at times by unhealthy or "neurotic" reasons in our responses to our children. We all are products of our past and present environment. We all have arrived at adulthood with certain twists in our personalities. These twists represent unhealthy needs that we use others to satisfy. And sometimes we use our children .

We should seek to overcome these undesirable motives as much as possible and seek in our discipline to satisfy our children's needs rather than our own. Thus, the basic motive behind discipline should not be to relieve our own frustration and anger, to satisfy our own ego needs for power, or to make ourselves look good but rather to help our children grow into responsible and responsive adults.

What Will My Child Learn from This Experience?

Every time a parent is faced with a situation requiring discipline, he or she should ask, *"What will my child learn from this experience?"* If the goal of discipline is to teach, then it is imperative that the parent know what he or she is trying to teach. Parents often inadvertently teach the child just the opposite of what they want him to learn.

> Bobby was suspected of being hyperactive at age four. Besides the usual characteristics, he had frequent temper tantrums. Although his poor emotional control made him prone to the tantrums, he was encouraged to continue by the way his family reacted to them.
>
> Bobby was the middle of three children. His big brother was ten and played little league baseball. His little sister was eighteen months old. Bobby didn't get much attention around the house—except when he had a tantrum. Then his father would try to "talk" him out of his tantrum. When this didn't work, he yelled and scolded. The scenes could go on for fifteen or twenty minutes. But on those few occasions when Bobby played quietly, no one ever talked or listened to him. He craved attention but got it only by misbehaving. He was actually being taught to have tantrums.

His parents were instructed to promptly place him in time out when he had a tantrum without saying anything except something like, "That kind of behavior isn't allowed in this house." On the other hand, they were encouraged purposely to give him wholesome attention throughout the day when he was engaged in acceptable behavior. In two weeks, his tantrums were virtually gone.

As in this case, parents often teach children the opposite of what they think they are teaching. They should frequently ask themselves, "What is my child learning from this experience?"

The First Step

"It's a lot easier to talk about discipline than it is to do it," a father exclaimed in a parent discussion group.

Of course he's right. It's one thing to talk in generalities about the ideals of child rearing; it's another to get down to the nitty-gritty of setting limits on your children's behavior. This is even truer when your child has a developmental disorder such as an attention deficit or learning disability. In this chapter, we will look at some practical ways of carrying out the ideals we so often talk about.

The first step in disciplining is deciding just what the rules will be in your family. This decision is one that each family must make for itself. The specific limits will not be the same for every family. The do's and don'ts will vary depending on many factors—where you live, your personalities, the personalities of your children, how many children are in the family, etc.

But each parent needs to decide definitely what the rules are to be. If your discipline is to be effective, your children must know what is expected of them. The line between acceptable and unacceptable behavior must be drawn firmly with a broad stroke so there is no doubt in the child's mind as to what is expected of him. Children feel much more secure when they know exactly where the boundaries and limits to their behavior lie.

The Behavior Traffic Light

A technique that helps parents to define their limits is what I call the *Behavior Traffic Light or BTL*. Using this technique, children's behavior can be compared to a traffic light. On this basis, behavior can be divided into three categories:

1. *Green or "Go" Behavior.*
Green represents behavior that is desired, approved, and encouraged. This is behavior that parents are heartily saying yes to.

Examples:

- The five-year-old who voluntarily puts her toys away.
- The seven-year-old who sits quietly and finishes his home work.
- The fourteen-year-old daughter who calls to tell you that she can't get home from school on time.
- The eight-year-old who finally is able to sit still without interrupting during the evening meal.
-

2. *Yellow or "Cautionary" Behavior.*

This is behavior that is tolerated for specific reasons, although it is not the ultimate behavior desired. This is behavior that really doesn't matter—behavior not important enough to quibble over or behavior that the parent cannot change anyway.

With ADHD kids, many examples of behavior fall into this category. There are many behaviors that are somewhat irksome to us but are not disruptive or destructive. Thus the cautionary behavior is behavior that we neither actively encourage nor discourage; we try to ignore it as best we can for now.

Examples:

- Fidgeting: The hyperactive child has restless arms and legs. If you try to stop this restlessness, much worse behavior will occur.
- Having to change play activities frequently. Due to the short attention span, they will need to change often.
- Need to talk: Their mind jumps from one thing to another. They need frequent opportunities to express themselves, and we must be patient to listen as they put their ideas together.

3. *Red or "No" Behavior.*

No behavior is behavior that is specifically disapproved of, behavior to which the parent is emphatically saying no. I suggest that parents must flash the red light to their children's behavior for the following reasons:

a. *When the child's behavior is a danger to himself or others.*
   Examples:
   - The two-year-old playing in the street.
   - The six-year-old playing with matches.

b. *When the child's behavior infringes on the rights of others.*
   Examples:
   - Interrupting Mother and Dad while they are talking.
   - Playing in the neighbor's flowerbeds.
   - Jumping up and down and running around in the den while the rest of the family is trying to watch TV or talk.

c. *When the child's behavior goes beyond the accepted morals, laws, or ethics of the community.*
   Examples:
   - The six-year-old who yells obscenities when he is angry.
   - The ten-year-old stealing a piece of candy from the neighborhood grocery.

d. *When the child's behavior is in direct defiance of the parents' authority.*
   Examples:
   - When the child looks at us and says emphatically no to a direct command from us.
   - When the child continues to deliberately violate a limit we have established.

Firmness and Confidence

Once parents have decided what the limits are, they should enforce them with firmness and confidence. Limits must be stated in such a way that only one message comes through: "These rules are real. I mean business." If the child senses uncertainty on the part of the parent(s), or if the limits shift from day to day, the line between acceptable and unacceptable behavior becomes not a solid line but a blur.

Parents need to realize that when they firmly set their limits, their children will not necessarily like them at that moment. Parents need to be secure enough in their role that this rebellion does not threaten them. When Janie screams, "I hate you," or Billy cries, "You're mean, you don't love me," it takes a real sense of security to refrain from caving in or acting hurt. But if parents stand their ground, their children will be the better for it.

Children are constantly testing limits. They do this for many reasons. Sometimes they are simply asking, "Who's the boss, you or me?" In this case, the parent needs to let the child know without a doubt who is boss. Sometimes the child genuinely is testing to find out just where the limits are. Parents can spell them out and write them down, but children still must find out for themselves just where the boundaries lie. And they do not learn from just one experience; they may have to test repeatedly until they are convinced the limits are solid. This certainly is true for the ADHD child.

Sometimes parents ask themselves, "Will they ever learn?" But they should not give up. Being consistent can be exasperating, but the only way the children ever will learn is by the parents "hanging in there" day in and day out.

Parents need to realize that their child with ADHD has more difficulty in learning the limits and staying within the boundaries. They should not be alarmed by this continued testing; it is natural.

Behavior Molding

Once parents have decided what the limits are, how do they go about enforcing them? Earlier we said the basic goal of discipline is to teach—to help the child learn appropriate information about life, his responsibilities, and his relationships to other people. So the parent must use effective teaching methods and techniques when it comes to the actual practice to enforcing limits. The parent needs a way to "mold" the child's behavior to fit the standards and limits they have set.

All of one's actions and behavior is directed at accomplishing certain goals. In the lives of children, the strongest driving forces are their needs for acceptance (by their parents), a feeling of security, a sense of worth, and an opportunity to grow and express their budding curiosity. As soon as they are born, children are learning which actions produce good feelings and which get bad feelings. Actions or behavior that fail to serve their purposes are soon dropped, and behavior that gets them good feelings or that is rewarded, is continued.

Unfortunately, the ADHD child's disorganized state "derails" his efforts to reach these goals. He still has the same goals as others, but he simply cannot work toward them as effectively. His uncontrolled and disorganized behavior is constantly leading him into situations and conflicts that produce bad feelings rather than good feelings for him.

Thus, as a child explores his world, his behavior is positively reinforced (i.e., rewarded) or negatively reinforced (i.e., punished). This process is constantly going on, and by this the child learns various lessons depending on how his behavior is reinforced. All behavior, good or bad, is learned in this way. It can be unlearned or extinguished in the same way. Undesirable behavior is likely to persist when, in the child's eyes, it pays off. But remember, it is what pays off in the child's eyes that counts, not what seems to be best to us.

For example, most of us as adults believe that a spanking would be unpleasant and unrewarding to a child. But this was not true for eight-year-old Albert. His father was gone most of the time on business trips, and his mother was all wrapped up in social and civic activities. Albert received very little attention except when he did mischievous things like writing on the wall with crayons. Even though each time he did this he got a spanking and a scolding, he persisted in doing it. To Albert the pain of the spanking was worth the coveted reward of parental attention, which he could get only by misbehaving.

The Tools of Discipline: Behavior-Molding Techniques

If the goal of discipline is to teach, the first step is to decide what we want our children to learn, thus the process of setting limits discussed already. The next step is the true test of our parental piloting skills: that's the point at which we ask, "Now that I know what I want for my child, how do I reach this goal?" In other words, what do we use to turn the rudder of our child's personality in the direction of maturity and self-discipline?

It is easy for us to fumble the controls at this point. If we use ineffective techniques, we can easily encourage the very behavior we are trying to eliminate. To avoid this error when faced with a disciplining decision, we need to ask ourselves another very important question. This key question is, "How do I do it?" Or in other words, *"How do I help my child to learn from this experience?"*

The next step is to learn how to use the rudder of discipline to direct the child's behavioral engine in the direction we as parents want it to go so our child will learn what we want him or her to learn.

Clay in the Hands of the Potter

Earlier we said that the basic goal of discipline is to teach. So when we come to the act of setting limits, and thus directing the child's energies, we need methods that effectively teach what we want the child to learn. Such effective techniques will help us "mold" the child's behavior toward the goals, or destinations, we have set.

When a potter is creating a work of art, he does not set the wet mound of clay on the potter's wheel, give it one or two slaps with his hands, and proclaim "It is done!" as he stands back to admire his work.

Instead, the creation of a work of art is a rather tedious process. The essential word here is *"process."* Time and effort are the key ingredients. The potter sets the wheel turning and then laboriously works the clay with his hands, gradually molding it into the shape of a symmetrical, balanced work of art.

In the same sense, we do not instantly produce mature individuals from the immature clay our children represent. Our children do not become what we want them to be by our simply wishing it, or by our telling them what we expect, or by our whacking them on the bottom a few times. Rather, we effectively discipline by molding their behavior as the potter molds the clay. We direct and reward behavior in small steps, painstakingly and slowly, as we mold our children through a daily process toward the ultimate goal of maturity by using effective teaching tools.

The techniques of discipline we will consider in detail in this chapter are not new. Parents have been using these methods in one way or another since the beginning of the family. We are simply putting a name on them and showing how they can be rightly applied to contemporary situations faced by today's parents.

Learning is going on all the time as an individual—child or adult—interacts with the environment. Behavior, and eventually ideals and desires, are modified, molded, or steered by three primary mechanisms or processes. These become our tools of discipline.

These tools are:

1. Instruction
2. Example or modeling
3. Enforced consequences
   - natural consequences
   - logical consequences
   - positive reinforcement
   - negative reinforcement

We will now look at each of these tools in some detail.

Instruction

Communicating clearly to the child what is expected of him is absolutely necessary for effective discipline. This is particularly true for the child with ADHD, who is not always tuned in to us to begin with.

Signals are verbal and non-verbal techniques we parents use to inform and guide our children. A good signal is one that unmistakably captures the child's attention and in the process conveys to the child what is expected of him as well as what the consequences of proper or improper behavior will be. Parents usually use such signals without being aware of the process.

Signals, in the form of *physical prompts*, are frequently necessary with young children. For example, if we want a young child to sit in his chair and eat, we may pick him up and place him in the chair. If a toddler starts to tear a magazine, we take it out of his hands, lift him away from the coffee table, and sit him in the middle of the floor. We are non-verbally saying, "You are not allowed to play with the magazine on the coffee table. You are allowed to play in the middle of the floor with this old one." Obviously many degrees of physical force can be involved in this. Certainly the force should be appropriate for the situation and not be overbearing or harsh.

More often, we use *verbal prompts* as signals. These signals should not come as threats, warnings, or bribes. Such negative signals are not only ineffective; they may even increase undesirable behavior. One common example of this type of self-defeating signal is to say to a misbehaving child, "If I've told you once I've told you a million times …"

Consider what is actually being communicated to the child. The statement, of course, expresses the parent's frustration and perhaps anger, but it rarely changes behavior in any constructive direction. From the child's point of view, no consequence for his behavior has been experienced. With such signals, the child perceives that he can repeat the defiant behavior without risking unpleasant consequences. This brings up an important point. By giving a signal that does not lead to effective consequences, the parent reveals that he or she is dealing from a position of weakness rather than strength.

Verbal signals, to be most effective, should not be negative or self-defeating. They should clearly state in words and tone the child can understand what is expected. Contrary to what many parents seem to think, their verbal directives or commands do not control their child's behavior. It is the consequence implied by the verbal signal that affects behavior. We can see why it is so important that verbal signals—whether they be demands, reprimands, or whatever—be backed up by relatively immediate and consistent consequences.

An essential part of discipline is this process of signaling to our children our wishes and limits—our behavioral goals. But the process of instruction involves more than signals. The growing human mind is a factual sponge. Children are compulsive absorbers of data—facts, impressions, feelings, meanings. In all times and places they are asking, "What, when, who, why, and how?" They want to learn. As we nurture this hunger for knowledge, we are helping our children acquire a knowledge base from which to make rational decisions about the world and how they fit into it. The right facts will help them understand how the world works and how their behavior elicits positive and negative consequences: "See, fire is hot. It burns!"

This factual input, if clear and consistent, will help our children mature more appropriately and become more effective at self-discipline.

Example or Modeling

The process of modeling desired behavior is one of the most direct ways our children learn. This learning by example is something we and our children do every day—most of the time unconsciously, other times deliberately. We model attitude, emotional control, and sense of responsibility primarily in this non-deliberate but certain manner.

Our children learn how to eat, bathe, dress, and brush their teeth by observing us. By saying "thank you" when someone does a favor for us, we lead our children do the same. If we live up to our promises, they are more likely to act responsibly. Indeed, much of our children's behavior is "caught" by means of such indirect modeling. At other times, our modeling will be much more direct.

When we began teaching our son at about age four to make up his bed, his mother actively used modeling. She introduced him to the idea by saying, "I think you are old enough to make your bed. Let's see how to do it." She then spent time with him demonstrating techniques of bed making. This was done in an enthusiastic and positive manner. After working together sufficiently so that he was quite familiar with the procedure, she then said, "I bet you can make you bed by yourself. Let me see how well you can do it." As he attempted the task, he was encouraged and praised. As he grew older, more exact methods were demonstrated.

A few years later, she used this same technique with effectiveness to teach our daughter to make her bed. Using this same general technique, our children were taught to keep their room clean, mow the lawn, set the table, and talk politely.

Parents usually do not see this modeling as a form of discipline. But in truth, it is one of our most effective tools available to us. Using it wisely avoids the need for more negative measures to unlearn bad habits later.

Enforced Consequences

Behavior is changed or modified by the consequences elicited by that behavior. Behavior that produces what the person perceives as positive consequences—gets him what he wants or makes him feel good—is likely to be continued. Behavior that elicits painful consequences is likely to attenuate and become less dominant. In this sense, consequences are our primary teachers.

All behavior has results and consequences, and these consequences themselves send definite messages back to us, the actor of the behavior. These messages inevitably modify how we act in the future. The judicious use of behavioral consequences is one of the more potent discipline techniques available to parents.

Consequences come in several forms. The ones that are important to us as we discuss discipline are these:

- natural consequences
- logical consequences
- positive reinforcement (rewards)
- negative reinforcement (punishment)

Now let's look at each of these.

Natural Consequences

Natural consequences are those imposed by nature—that is, by the inherent quality of the behavior itself. When a child experiences natural consequences, he or she is learning by trial and error. Some examples of natural consequence are: touching a hot stove and getting burned; forgetting your lunch and going hungry; spending your allowance on candy and having none left for the toy you wanted to buy; starting a fight with someone twice your size and getting banged up.

Trial and error is an effective form of learning. We learn much of what we know about life in this manner. Our children certainly need the opportunity to learn from their own successes and failures.

No doubt, nature is teaching us all the time. A wise parent will evaluate the circumstances and refrain, when possible, from interfering with the child's experience of nature's laws at work. But as parents, we do walk a fine line at this point.

For example, when Susan's son got in the habit of chronically forgetting his lunch, she repeatedly made an inconvenient trip to school to drop it off for him. In frustration, she asked me about this. I suggested that she quit taking the lunch for him when he forgot it. "But he will go hungry," she worried. I assured her that skipping lunch occasionally would not cause any bodily harm.

Susan was expressing the usual and natural concern of parents. Actually, her angry badgering of her son was doing more psychological harm than any one day's hunger would ever do. Once she got up the courage to let him experience this natural consequence (i.e., going hungry), her son forgot his lunch only two more times. From then on, he always remembered.

Logical Consequences

Certainly we must protect our children from much that nature would impose. We cannot always let nature take her natural course because the results would be harmful. It is at this point that logical consequences come into play. Logical consequences are similar to natural consequences except that they are subtly conditioned by the parent rather than imposed by nature. To work effectively, these consequences must logically relate to the behavior in question.

Let's look at some examples:

> Eight-year-old Jimmy continues to bounce his basketball in the house after his mother has requested he not do so. She quietly takes the basketball and puts it on the closet shelf. "You cannot play with your ball until tomorrow," she states.

This is a logical consequence of Jimmy's behavior: "You play with your ball in an improper way and you will lose the privilege of using it." Logical consequences, to be effective, must be logical; they should not be artificial or out of proportion to the offense.

> Seven-year-old Matthew spills his milk at the dinner table. Punishment says, "Gee, Matt, you're so clumsy. When are you going to learn to hold a glass?"

Logical consequences say, "It seems like you've made a mess. Here's a sponge to clean it up." The child already feels bad, and there is nothing to be gained by making him feel worse. But by the use of logical consequences, the parent quietly but certainly conveys to the child the message that making messes carries consequences. You have to clean them up.

> Nine-year-old Susan wants to go to Tricia's house to play, but she has left her toys and clothes strewn all over her room. Mother responds, "Sorry, you can't go out until your room is clean."

Logical consequence: you can't do what you want to until your responsibilities are carried out.

> A sixteen-year-old wants to use the family car. A requirement is that, through chores and odd jobs, he earns enough money for gas. If he doesn't earn the money, no car.

Logical consequences should be applied with a minimum of yelling, screaming, and harsh words. Such attention-giving methods negate the value of the logical consequences. The purpose is to help the child see clearly that dependable consequences follow behavior in a natural, logical manner. Further, he can learn that he can control the consequences by altering or controlling his behavior.

Positive Reinforcement or Rewards

One of the most effective ways of molding, or directing, our children's behavior is by means of positive reinforcement. This requires us to take note of our children's desirable or "go" behavior, acknowledge it, and reward it.

Rewards and reinforcements may come in many forms. Some parents effectively use privileges, money, points, or other material items as rewards. Such material rewards may, or may not, work well for a given child or in a given situation. There are specific instances, however, where material rewards of various kinds are indicated. Some of these will be discussed later.

Parents, however, must not overlook the most effective, yet the most inexpensive, positive reward of all: that of genuine attention. Children, like adults, constantly seek to satisfy their need for love, social acceptance, and self-respect. Praise, particularly when given in front of other children, is an extremely strong motivational tool. Children are on a continual search for attention. They will do almost anything to gain personal recognition. Recognizing and responding to this need is one powerful way we steer our children's behavior toward the goals we have set.

As mentioned earlier, parents can unconsciously reward the very behavior they want to eliminate. They do so by responding to the child only when he misbehaves.

> Three-year-old Cathy still wets her pants. Every time she does it, her mother spanks her, yells, and argues—for about ten minutes. When Cathy goes for hours without wetting, her mother never says anything.

In this situation, Cathy is rewarded for wetting her pants with attention. A child would rather be thought of as stupid or obnoxious than not be thought of at all.

> Mrs. Jones is cooking dinner. Sammy asks for a cookie. "No," his mother replies. "It's too close to mealtime." Sammy begins to whine and cry. "Will you hush," she yells, but he keeps on crying. Finally, in frustration she says, "Well just this once. Now will you go away and be quiet?"

Sammy's whining and crying has been positively rewarded. The next time he wants a cookie, he knows what to do: just whine and cry long enough and Mother will give in.

Here are some healthy ways we can use positive reinforcement in molding our child's behavior:

a. *Recognition*
Recognition from family, friends, teachers, and other important people serves as a strong motivator. This may be done in many ways:

- "Billy, I am so pleased that you were able to put your pants on by yourself."
- "Wally, you tied your shoes by yourself."
- "Sean, you made an A on your math test."

b. *Encouragement*

We all, children and adults, need to be encouraged.

- "You are trying very hard to make your bed. You can do it so well."
- "That was a super effort you made in the football game."

c. *Praise*

Genuine praise for a job well done or a good effort extended is one of the greatest motivators.

- "I appreciate the good job you did cleaning the yard."
- "I was very pleased by the way you acted while we were visiting Grandmother's house."

d. *Sense of accomplishment*

The knowledge that one has done a job well or learned something significant is itself a powerful motivating force.

e. *Material gain*

The chance of personal gain is a definite human motivating factor, although it is not always the most important. The knowledge that desirable actions on his part will get him something he wants, such as treats, money, or time, can be strong reinforcer for a particular child. As discussed previously, rewards, to be effective, must be immediate and tangible to the child.

It does little good to tell a third grader that if she makes straight A's she will get a bicycle at the end of the year—or that she will get a dollar for every A she has on her report card. Such a goal is too distant and intangible for most children.

More appropriately we could say, "Susan, complete the first five problems of your homework now, and then you can take a break and have a cookie and juice." You give a small, immediate reward for one small step in the right direction and then repeat this process over and over.

We should reward each little step toward the right goal, not wait to give one big reward for total perfection. As learning is reinforced, the material becomes more and more indelibly imprinted on the conscious and subconscious mind of the child.

Many ideas for reinforcers will come to mind. Some things are already reinforcing to a child right from the start—food, warmth, and cuddling, for example. Babies do not have to learn that these are desirable; they are desirable because they meet basic needs. Such automatic reinforcers are called natural reinforcers because they do not have to be learned. Most reinforcers are not natural; they are learned. Money, music, mother's voice, flowers, and friends are all learned reinforcers. They are reinforcing because children have learned that these objects or events are desirable and give pleasure.

What is most rewarding or reinforcing to a given child will depend a great deal on what that child has learned to like. But we should always remember that the most potent reward we have is genuine appreciation and honest attention for desirable behavior.

However, take note. Recent research points out that it is possible to "overpraise" a child. If a parent or caretaker is continually handing out praise, it loses its punch. Also, praise should be genuine. In other words, find something worthy of praise before mindlessly saying, "You are a good boy." This brings up another point. Praise should always be directed to the action, the behavior at hand, not aimed at the person. Praise the action, not the person. "You tried very hard. I am proud of your effort," is a healthy praise.

Negative Reinforcement or Punishment

Some childcare specialists insist that punishment has no place at all in today's child rearing. Having worked with families in a variety of environments as well as parenting two children of my own to maturity, I know that punishment has a necessary place in discipline. But the use of punishment should be kept in perspective. My experience suggests that we parents should aim at a positive balance in our relationships with our children in which we use positive methods most of the time, with negative reinforcement or punishment constituting less of our interactions. This is a desirable goal, and I believe it is an attainable one.

The most potent punishment in my experience is some form of logical consequences. "You haven't cleaned your room, so you cannot go out and play." For the younger child, isolation and deprivation of parental attention for fairly short periods of time are useful negative reinforcers. This kind of "time-out" procedure works well for the younger child.

Nagging, yelling, and threatening are not only ineffective, but they also eventually backfire.

> The family is watching TV. But four-year-old Shannon continues to jump up, stand in front of others, and talk loudly, although he has been asked not to do so.

Appropriate discipline or negative reinforcement would be for his father to say firmly but quietly, "Shannon, I asked you not to interfere with the others. Go to your room until this program is over."

My experience suggests that such negative reinforcement must have a place in the family—but only when coupled with a heavy dose of positive reinforcement for acceptable behavior.

Spanking

While spanking can be a proper and effective discipline tool at times, it can be misused. Applied too frequently or too harshly, spanking can provoke anger and rebellion. Inappropriate spanking overexcites the child and makes him less open to learning and change. I tell parents who frequently use spanking that they are using their major cannons to fight minor skirmishes. When it comes to a real crucial battle, they do not have any weapons left with which to make their point. Spanking should not be used as an emotional pop-off value for parental frustration. Such use of spanking as an outlet for our anger and frustration is not only ineffective in changing the child's behavior, but it can also lead to the parent losing control.

In general, spanking is not a very practical tool to use with children with ADHD. It only tends to over-stimulate them and leads to more loss of control. While is it extremely important for parents to set firm limits for children with ADHD, these limits need to be enforced in deliberate but unemotional ways.

Using "I" and "You" Statements

One of the most effective, tools in parent-child communication is the practice of using "*I*" statements instead of "*you*" statements. Since these are new terms to many, it might help to clarify the meaning of "I" and "you" statements.

"You" Statements

"You" statements sound something like this:

"You're late again today."
"Can't you do anything right?"
"You're so messy."
"You just don't try to do what I ask."
"You're lazy."
"You never do your chores."
"You never hand in your work on time."
"Why are you always getting into trouble?"
"You're late again with that project?"

Such "you" statements are by nature accusatory and negating. They put the recipient on the defensive because he or she feels attacked and threatened. The innate reflex when one feel threatened is to emotionally gear up for a defense. Under such circumstances, one's intellectual resources, attention, and energies are focused on defending oneself, one's integrity, and one's ego. When one is in such a defensive posture, one is not receptive to learning, change, or growth. So when "you" statements are used to correct a child, they create such a negative emotional cloud that learning is thwarted. Once the child has been accused or attacked, he "hears" little else that is said. The negative feelings engendered likely will not go away quickly. These negative feelings, in turn, interfere with ongoing relationships.

"I" Statements

"I" statements, on the other hand, are simple statements about how another's behavior or actions affect us or make us feel. Rather than attack the other person, "I" statements matter-of-factly inform the child or other person how his or her behavior, positive or negative, affects us. Done in a nonthreatening, non-accusatory way, these "I" statements are more likely to enlist respect and corrective action.

Something in our human nature makes us, children and adults, responsive to the honesty of "I" statements. Since we are not on the defensive, we are free to listen and change.

"I" statements sound something like this:

> "I am frustrated when I see your room in such a mess."
> "I must work harder when you forget to take out the trash."
> "My ears hurt when you shout so loud. I would appreciate your keeping it a little quieter."
> "I get nervous when I don't know that you are going to be late from school."
> "I am happy that you remembered to take out the trash."
> "I like this meal."
> "I am excited that you made an A in math."
> "I am pleased with the way you have been making your bed and cleaning your room."
> "I am disappointed that you would deliberately disobey me."
> "I like the way you were polite to your aunt today."
> "I don't like to hear you yell at your sister."

The Value of "I" Statements

The use of such "I" statements facilitate communication in the family in several ways:

"I" statements reduce the amount of blaming and nagging we do. "I" statements do not blame. They state facts. Nagging creates hard feelings and repressed resentment, which tends to lead to an ever-deepening spiral of antagonistic behavior within a family. The more we can get away from such blaming and nagging, the more likely our homes are to be pleasant, nurturing places for all of us.

"I" statements are excellent teaching tools. Remember, the essence of discipline is teaching. In my experience, children who are surrounded by "I" statements learn to use them to facilitate their own communication of feelings.

Since they are based on facts, "I" statements reduce the amount of defensive feelings and behavior in the child or other person, thus leaving an open door for the person to do something about the fact, situation, or behavior that is bothering us, the sender of the message. The child can change his behavior or correct a condition without losing face or personal prestige.

"I" statements also serve as a nonthreatening, legitimate way to express one's emotions. Feelings and emotions, both positive and negative, need to be expressed. "I" statements allow us to express our emotions in such a way that others can know exactly how we feel and why. With anger, frustration, hurt, they allow us to get our feelings out in the open without inciting additional negative feelings in the receiver.

For those who have never tried them, "I" statements may at first take some effort. Their use may seem a little strange, or at least a little artificial. But if you try using them for a while, you will find that, more and more, they come easily and unconsciously. You will also see what a difference they can make in your relationships with your loved ones.

Communication of Negative Feelings—Anger, Hurt, and Disappointment—in the Family

Relationships at home and at school are often poisoned by our inability to deal with negative emotions, such as anger and frustration.

This is very true for children with ADHD and those who must live with them. Negative interactions take up so much of our time because we do not know how to handle negative emotions in healthy, constructive ways. Certainly we cannot live in close contact with each other without getting angry, hurt, frustrated, and disappointed—all is not roses, ice cream, and chocolate chip cookies. When they do bubble to the surface, negative emotions need attention. To repress or bury our negative feelings only results in more hurt.

Anger is one emotion, for example, that most of us have trouble with. It is one of the most difficult emotions to understand and control. Some people, when angry, have tantrums and send everyone around them, friend and foe alike, scurrying for cover. Others in the face of their anger maintain a stoic, icy silence, not openly letting their feelings be known. They may sulk, pout, or simply tighten up their facial muscles, staring with eyes of steel. Both of these extremes of emotional expression are unhealthy: uncontrolled outbursts of anger destroy a lot of property, break teeth, and start large and small wars.

But holding in one's anger is just as damaging. Seething, bottled-up anger leads to ulcers, headaches, heart attacks, and if nothing else, nasty dispositions. Unfortunately, many people have not been able to find a happy medium between these extremes.

Healthy, productive ways of dealing with anger do exist. If we can learn to handle our own anger properly and in turn, teach this to our children, our families will have much smoother sailing now; our children will have a much happier, healthier lives in the future.

Healthy expression of negative feelings requires three steps:

- First, we need to *claim the feeling.*
- Second, we must *name the feeling.*
- Third, we must properly *aim the feeling.*

With this process, we get our feelings out in the open in an honest way. In doing this, we can make statements like this:

"I am angry."
"I feel frustrated."

"I feel cheated that you are going hunting on our anniversary."

We claim the feeling by saying, "I am angry," rather than saying, "You make me angry." We are also honestly verbalizing exactly what we feel. We name the feeling by saying, "I feel angry" rather than, "You really don't care about me." Then we aim our feelings at the proper target by stating why we are angry. "I feel angry because you are an hour late in getting home." Too often we are angry at one thing or person but aim it at someone or something else.

As you may have realized by now, this technique of handling negative emotions is a practical application of "I" statements we discussed previously.

Practice Being the Parent

Some parents hesitate to exert their authority for fear of hurting their child's feelings or warping him psychologically. I hope that by now you are convinced that it is the undisciplined child who is in danger, not the properly disciplined one. I have found to my initial surprise that opportunity for real communication, instruction, and understanding between me and my children often occurs soon after I have exerted my authority. Deep down, the child senses a need for limits, protection, and discipline. When these are in place in his life, he is a more secure, ultimately happier person.

So indeed, discipline is not something we parents do to our children; it is something we do for them.

For Thought and Discussion

1. The use of instruction.

    a. How clearly do you use instruction with your child?

    b. Are your signals readily understood by him or her? Do you often send mixed signals?

2. The use of modeling and example.

    a. What are some ways you have used example to encourage good behavior in your child?

    b. What is one negative habit or behavior you have encouraged in your child by example?

3. Using logical consequences.

    a. Have you ever tried to use logical consequences before? Did the effort work?

    b. Can you think of a current behavior that you might modify using logical consequences? Develop a plan.

4. Using positive reinforcement

    a. Have you tried using rewards before?

    b. List at least five things for each of your children that would be rewarding to them.

    c. List at least three desirable traits or behaviors presently exhibited by your child that you could reinforce and encourage.

5. Applying negative reinforcement.

    a. What forms of punishment have you used in the past?

    b. How successful have these methods been?

6. Review the following situations. What discipline technique would be most effective?

Instruction
Example or modeling
Logical consequences
Positive reinforcement
Negative reinforcement

    a. A four-year-old who eats very little at meals and then keeps asking for snacks
    b. A five-year-old who repeatedly disobeys while you

are shopping

c. A fourth-grader who fails to bring home his homework assignments

d. A six-year-old who hits his classmate when provoked

e. A seventh-grader who fails math

f. A first-grader who talks out of turn

g. A first-grader who continues to interrupt

h. A ten-year-old who has a hard time keeping his room organized and neat

7. Review the discussion of the behavioral traffic light.

a. List three desirable or "go" behaviors you would like your child to exhibit:

b. List three undesirable or "no" behaviors you would like to see your child stop:

CHAPTER NINE

Strategies for a Healthy Self-Image

Who Do You Think You Are?

"WHO do you think you are?"

This question is often spoken in jest or scorn. It is, however, a question deserving serious attention. The answer can determine the course of one's life.

As researchers in medicine and psychology have probed the depths of the human personality, they have affirmed the crucial place one's self-image plays in determining what kind of person one will be. What one thinks of himself or herself plays the biggest role in determining the limits of one's potential.

The Importance of the Self-image

I didn't learn to swim until I was an adult. For some reason, I had a desperate fear of water. As a growing youngster, I had no self-confidence around a body of water larger than a mud puddle. Even in my high school swim class, I could hardly bring myself to turn loose of the side of the swimming pool. I simply had no faith in my ability to stay afloat. I knew I would sink!

When I was in college, I told a friend that I wanted to learn to swim.

"Look," he counseled, "half the battle in learning to swim is believing that you will not sink. As long as you have no confidence in yourself, you will never learn."

He taught me to tread water and to float. Then he pushed me into water over my head. I timidly began to move my arms. As I learned that I could stay afloat, I began to believe I could really swim. And I was soon swimming.

My experience is a parable of life. One's self-image determines the limits of one's accomplishments. We can, and will, do what we think we can. One inevitably becomes the kind of person one believes oneself to be. We can swim in the arena of life only as we believe that we can stay afloat. We become what we think ourselves to be.

We can expand this to say that children have a remarkable way of living up to the expectations of the important adults in their lives. What we think of our children will inevitably influence what they really are.

> Byron, a fourteen-year-old, was brought to me because he was failing in school. Throughout the elementary grades, he had trouble with reading and math, and he was retained in the second grade. Now in the seventh grade he was failing almost all of his subjects. Both parents were frustrated and unhappy with his performance. They did not have any idea why he was a poor student. In periods of desperation, they had said things like, "I don't know why you are so dumb."

> At the first visit, I asked Byron's mother if she thought his intelligence was low, normal, or high.

> "Probably not very high," she responded.

> When I talked to Byron, he was sad and depressed. I asked him the same question. "I guess I'm just dumb," he replied.

> Surprisingly, however, he was neither dumb nor stupid. His IQ was 125, which was well above the normal range. But other tests showed that

he had a mild attention deficit and receptive language disability. The subtle dysfunctions hampered his efficiency in academic work. Because of these unrecognized problems, he had become progressively behind in school. By the seventh grade, his underachievement was complicated by his poor self-image and feelings of inadequacy. He had inevitably absorbed the expectations of his parents and teachers and become a "failure" in his own eyes.

Byron's story is not all that rare. As I evaluate children with learning disabilities, I find that many, like Byron, are programmed to fail by the expectations of others.

We do become what we think ourselves to be.

The woman who thinks herself beautiful will indeed appear more beautiful, if for no other reason than because she cultivates and cares for what beauty she does possess. The student who thinks he can work the math problem will indeed try extra hard to live up to this image of himself. The one who thinks he is stupid in math is likely to quit trying before trying all the possibilities. One of the secrets of a successful teacher is knowing how to plant within the students a confidence that will keep them trying, never giving up on themselves.

A Balanced, Healthy Self-Image

A healthy self-image is one that leads the individual to accept himself or herself as a person of value and worth.

Let me illustrate what I mean by this:

Dr. Thomas Harris in his book, *I'M OK, You're OK*[5], states that there are four basic perspectives from which we can face life. These are:

"I'm not OK—you're OK."
"I'm not OK—you're not OK."
"I'm OK—you're not OK."
"I'm OK—you're OK."

The first life perspective, *"I'm not OK—you're OK,"* is probably the most common. Such individuals have an inferiority complex.

---

5   Harris, Thomas, *I'm OK, You're OK.* New York: Harpers, 1969, 43.

They cannot see their own gifts and strengths. They see only their weaknesses.

This is often the self-image of the child with ADHD or learning disabilities. They feel inferior to others. This insecurity leads to one of two protective mechanisms. Some cower in a corner, refusing to take any initiative for fear of failing. On the other hand, many people with such an inferiority complex take on the facade of aggressive assertion to compensate for their sense of inadequacy. Whatever means they use to compensate, people with an inferiority complex are basically unhappy and insecure.

Byron in our previous illustration is an example of this life perspective.

The second perspective, *"I'm not OK—you're not OK,"* is indeed a warped one. Such an individual sees very little good in the world. He sees very little value in himself as well as in others.

> James was physically abused by his parents as a small child. By the time he was a preadolescent, he had a hard emotional shell that no one could break through. He seemed insensitive to all pain, his own as well as that of others. He was unable to get close to anyone. He grew up to be a very unhappy person.

A learning disabled child who meets nothing but failure and criticism is in danger of growing into such a warped self-hood.

The third life perspective, *"I'm OK—you're not OK,"* is also unhealthy. This perspective is distorted so the individual sees himself or herself as the center of their world.

> As a toddler, Becky had temper tantrums, and her parents gave in to all her demands. As a first grader, she could sweet talk her father into anything she wanted. She was showered with things. At school she was a bully, and she tried to manipulate her teacher the same way as she manipulated her parents. Consequently, she had few friends. As she grew older, she became more sullen and difficult to live with.

The fourth life perspective, "I'm OK—you're OK," is the one we seek for ourselves and for our children. When our children can look out on the world and say, "I'm OK and you're OK," we know they are healthy, whole individuals who have the fundamentals necessary for a happy life. This is the balanced self-image that will permit our children to reach their total potential.

This is the life perspective that will allow our children to love, live, and leave: to love others as they love themselves, to love life freely, making the most of their God-given talents, and to eventually be able to leave—emotionally and physically—the protective cocoon of the home and become a self-disciplining, self-motivated adult.

Yes, *love, live, leave* ... This is our ultimate goal for our children.

Special Problems of the Child with ADHD and Learning Disabilities

Helping the child with ADHD to grow up with a balanced sense of self-worth requires care and effort by all who impact his life. At every turn, the child is met with situations that tend to tear down and warp the self-image. Among these are the following.

1. *From an early age, he finds himself in constant conflict with the limits placed on him by parents, teachers, and other authority figures.* Since much of the behavior producing this conflict is not purposeful disobedience on his part, he is confused and frustrated. He gets the message, "There must be something wrong with me. I can't do anything right!"

2. *Lack of achievement in school reinforces the sense of being abnormal and inferior.* A child who sees himself getting further and further behind his peers in achievement easily loses his self-confidence. If this continues long enough, he may come to say, "Why try? I'm no good anyway."

3. *The child who is uneven in his development and who has significant discrepancies in his abilities may be confused by the contrast between what he can do easily and that which requires an inordinate amount of effort for rather minimal achievement.* He may be puzzled as he tries to understand what his capacities really are. The amount of study, including testing, that is needed in the diagnosis of a learning disability also can create

worry about himself. The child and his parents may be the victims of professionals disagreeing about diagnosis and treatment.

4. *The child may be jealous of other children and siblings for whom achievement comes easily.* There may be problems around school work at home, particularly if his brothers and sisters degrade him in any way for his less-than-perfect work. He may hear from school personnel or family the fallacy, "If you just work harder, you can do better." The child may be upset by the kinds of work he must do because of his disability: for example, a fourth-grade boy cried because he was doing the same kind of work his first-grade sister was doing.

5. *Poor coordination resulting in unsuccessful performance on the playground is also detrimental to the self-image.* Other children often ridicule the one who is poorly coordinated, and ridicule from a peer burns deeply.

What Can We Do?

While it can be difficult to overcome these problems, parents and professionals have some practical strategies to help the child retain a balanced sense of self-worth in spite of the odds:

1. *When the child breaks the rules or oversteps the limits, we should discipline firmly but kindly. We should aim the discipline at the offense and not at the child or his personality.*

The child should not be told, "Would you stop? You're nothing but trouble." Instead we might say, "Johnny, your jumping around is really bugging me. I think you should go to your room for fifteen minutes and see if you can stop." We then send him immediately to his room. If he doesn't go willingly and quickly, we take him by the shoulder and lead him to his room.

Rather than say, "Don't be stupid. I've told you that a hundred times," we should say something like, "I've explained that rule before. Please do what I asked."

Everyone should remember that one can discipline firmly without attacking the person or worth of the child.

2. *We should not punish the child for things he really cannot help, such as fidgeting or being clumsy.* (Remember yellow light behavior, as discussed in the previous chapter.)

3. *As much as possible, we should positively reinforce appropriate and desired behavior.* "Catch them being good and tell them so" is a healthy working motto. Always be on the lookout for the opportunity to honestly say something affirmative.

4. *If we suspect the child of having a behavior or learning problem, we should seek help as soon as possible so the proper diagnosis and treatment may be instituted.* Often such early intervention can circumvent much of the stress and conflict that blocks their success.

5. *We must seek an educational environment that treats the child as an individual,* recognizes his strengths and weaknesses, and helps him learn in his own way at a pace appropriate for his skills.

6. *We should help the child to discover his good qualities and superior skills.* All of us, even those with special problems, do have some good points and superior abilities. We all have a deep psychological need to excel in some area of life. Your child's hidden talent may be an isolated academic skill, a sport, a hobby, or music ability.

For instance, many children with ADHD are not very good at the traditional sports, such as football, basketball, and track, because of their lack of coordination. But often these children are quite well coordinated in water and are excellent swimmers. Thus swimming for fun and competition can be pursued as their area of excellence. One boy was a very poor reader but had perfect pitch and became a good musician in spite of his inability to read well.

7. *We should not use language that attacks the child's dignity or personal worth.* Children who are belittled as youngsters are likely to grow up with a poor self-image. They literally continue to belittle themselves throughout life. Such belittling adjectives as rude, ugly, stupid, or clumsy should not be used to describe children. Rude, stupid, ugly, etc., may be used to describe actions, if necessary, but they should not be used against the child himself. The danger is that the child may accept such an evaluation and make it a part of his self-image. If he thinks himself as rude, ugly, or stupid, he is likely, in the end, to behave that way. It is only natural for a rude boy to behave rudely.

Such precautions do not imply parents should not correct a child or criticize his behavior. There is, however, a big difference between criticizing the behavior and criticizing the child.

Rather than say, "You are a rude boy," a parent can say, "That was a rude thing to do. Apologize and go to your room." Such a statement is not an attack on the child's personality but does show disapproval of his behavior.

To the child who brings home a poor report card, a parent can say something like this: "Cathy, this doesn't look like you. I guess we will have to set up a regular homework time." To say, "I knew you were lazy, but I never expected this from a child of mine!" is to whittle away at the child's ego.

It is a hard lesson for us parents to remember, but discipline should be directed toward the misdeed and not toward the child's personality. Even if the child's personality leaves something to be desired, to attack it will only make it worse. Remember, we get a lot more out of a child, or anyone else, with positive reinforcement of good traits than we do by criticizing the undesirable traits.

What Are Healthy Expectations?

Just as dangerous as expecting too little of our children is expecting and demanding too much. Janie was a freckle-faced five-year-old with long auburn hair. She was brought to see me because of frequent crying spells, nightmares, bed wetting, and undisciplined behavior. The parents were quite concerned. "She won't sit still, she doesn't remember to feed her puppy, and she's not learning to read like the other kids in her kindergarten."

> Janie turned out to be a normal girl who was extremely frustrated. She was an only child, and neither of her parents had been around young children. They expected her to behave more like a ten-year-old than a five-year-old. Her inability to live up to these unrealistically high expectations frustrated both her and her parents and resulted in her emotional problems. The parents were encouraged to let Janie be a five-year-old. They were told that most five-year-old children don't learn to read and shouldn't be pushed to do so; neither are they likely to remember to do their chores without help; and they certainly can't sit still.

A child who is constantly pushed and badgered to perform or act beyond his level of maturity or capabilities is in danger of developing a distorted self-image. Every child has a basic drive to please and to be accepted by his parents. If he is constantly failing to live up to their expectations, he begins to wonder what is wrong. The average student who is pushed to make all A's begins to think himself stupid when he constantly fails to reach that mark—even though no one openly told him he was stupid. Such "inferiority complexes" frequently result when a child constantly fails to live up to unrealistic goals.

The opposite of this is the child who is overprotected and indulged. This child develops an exaggerated opinion of himself, which is just as much a distortion of his self-image as a belittled opinion of oneself. Such a child often grows up to expect from others the same overindulgence he received from his parents; or he may become bitter and disappointed when he finds out that he cannot live up to the exaggerated place in life his family has established for him.

No doubt children have a remarkable way of fulfilling the expectations of important adults in their lives. Parental expectations should be realistic and appropriate to the child's age and level of maturity. If parents expect too little, growth is hampered; and if they expect bad behavior, their prophecy may very well come true.

Parent-Child Relationships

Probably the oldest and still the most widely fought debate in child rearing is the one between those who feel that parents should be permissive and those who feel parents should be strict in their discipline. Let us look at the consequences of both of these extremes.

1. *Permissiveness.*

Extreme permissiveness is the attitude on the part of parents that allows the child unlimited freedom. The parent interferes with the child's life only as a last resort. In extreme over-permissiveness, limits are few or nonexistent. A child reared in such an environment may be creative, impulsive, energetic, aggressive, and independent. Certainly these can be—and often are—desirable traits. But he is also likely to have trouble controlling his impulses, lacks self-control, and has difficulty cooperating with others. Extreme permissiveness is likely to be more harmful than good. The child will have a hard time adjusting socially and conforming to the rules of society.

Parents may be overpermissive for several reasons. There are the sophisticated parents who adopt permissiveness because it seems to be the thing to do and it is what the experts recommend whether the parents are comfortable with this attitude or not. Other parents take the route of permissiveness because they lack confidence in themselves to the point that they cannot take the initiative needed to set rules and enforce them. Then there are those who are permissive out of guilt. They feel a need to atone for some fancied or real sin and do this by "taking it easy" on the child. This is all too frequently the subconscious motive of parents who have children with handicaps.

2. *Rigidity.*

The attitude of extreme rigidity and strictness is one in which the parent sets very narrow limits on the child's behavior. The child's life is hemmed in by a constant barrage of no's.

Extreme rigidity expects the child to be a "perfect angel," and when the child does not conform to this, he is severely punished.

Parents with this attitude tend to be perfectionists and expect the same of their children. The child is allowed little freedom to be a child—to be spontaneous, free, and happy. Children reared in homes with this attitude tend to be conformists, cooperative, quiet, passive, and self-controlled. They often have trouble making decisions for themselves because the decisions have always been made for them. Often a load of hostility is buried underneath their passivity because their own personality has been stifled for so long. And sometimes these children rebel against the rigidity and strictness of their home with vengeance.

Avoid Extremes

Either extreme permissiveness or extreme strictness is unhealthy for our children. Extremes in either direction tend to produce unhappy, angry children. Children in these circumstances are likely to have trouble understanding themselves and adjusting to society.

In the rigid relationship, the child's self-hood is squelched into almost nothingness by too many and too harsh rules; in the overly permissive relationship, the child's self-hood cannot developed due to lack of self-discipline.

The Eventual Goal: Self-Discipline

Discipline and self-control are necessary for a person to be a creative, successful adult. Each of us, adults and children, has the right to develop in his or her own way until doing so infringes on the rights of others. Thus limits on our behavior, from the outside or the inside, are necessary.

Our eventual goal as parents is for our children to develop a measure of self-discipline and self-control that allows them to express their creativity constructively but not be so overcontrolling that their originality is snuffed out.

A balanced attitude on our part as parents is needed. This attitude allows the child as much freedom and independence as he can handle while firmly setting limits on unhealthy behavior. The child should have freedom to be a child, to express his curiosity, and to try new things; but this freedom will have to be limited when it interferes with the rights of others or with his own safety.

Certainly, the child with ADHD often requires the setting and enforcing of limits much more consistently than with some other children. But even with the child with ADHD, we look forward to the time when his own internal self-control will mature and take charge.

Some Unhealthy Attitudes

Sometimes parents load the parent-child relationship with attitudes that create within the child almost continuous feelings of hurt and frustration. Often anger and rebellion are the results.

1. *Oversubmission* is the parental attitude by which parents capitulate to the child's every whim without regard to their rights as parents or the child's rights to grow.

Mrs. Gray complained about Tony's temper tantrums. She would try to soothe his rage with condescending talk, but this never succeeded. She would finally give up and let him have his way just to make peace.

When it was suggested that by giving in to his display of anger she was rewarding his rebellion, Mrs. Gray cried, "But what can I do?" It was recommended that she put Tony in time-out until the tantrum subsided. She winced, "But that would be so cruel." Mrs. Gray failed to understand that the real cruelty was in submitting to Tony's tantrums and thus teaching him that such behavior was a way to get what he wanted. By school age, Tony was an obnoxious child with no friends and poor grades because he tried to manipulate everyone like he did his mother.

2. *Punitiveness* is the parental attitude in which parents load the child with unrealistic restrictions, often in anger. Such punitiveness builds up a reservoir of frustration that periodically boils over in bad behavior, sneaking, stealing, or overt rebellion. Many juvenile delinquents come from homes where they are unfairly treated, with no regard for their rights.

3. *Rejection* is the parental attitude that gives the child no place in the family group. The child is wounded by an attitude that says, "You're a burden. I don't want you. I didn't want you in the first place." Such an attitude is not expressed in word so much as in actions. The child who has to live with this attitude is likely to be a brooding, lonely, and hostile child. He develops a storehouse of anger against life and those who have deprived him of the loving acceptance he sorely needs.

The child who is loved but not submitted to, who is disciplined but not repressed, will still express anger and rebellion, but it will be a healthy anger he can learn to control. The extremes of oversubmission, overprotection, and rejection produce deep-seated anger that is difficult to overcome and leaves a permanent mark.

Mutual Respect

The relationship between parent and child should be based on the same mutual respect that we would want to apply to all of our personal relationships. This does not mean that we should relax our goals or compromise our ideals for our children. But it does mean that we will treat our children as persons. When discipline is required, it will be given with firmness, purpose, and understanding but without anger, retaliation, or sarcasm. It means that we will treat our children with the same courtesy that we extend to adults and that we expect from the child.

Helping Siblings Cope

"Fights like brothers and sisters" is a common saying that reflects some of the ambivalence coloring sibling relationships. Yet these relationships are among the richest and most enduring bonds of life. Siblings typically spend more time with each other than with their parents. From birth on, they influence each other's social, emotional, and intellectual development in both positive and negative ways.

How is this significant relationship affected when one sibling has a major illness or developmental disability, such as ADHD? This important question is touched on by Debra Lobato, PhD, in an article in *Pediatric Management.*

She states, "Investigators are focusing on measures of potential psychological strength as well as weakness" in families where one sibling has a chronic health or developmental problem. She points out that a review of recent, carefully controlled studies suggests that a child's disability or illness may not directly influence a sibling's self-concept, self-esteem, social competence, or behavioral adjustment in a negative way. One study of college-age siblings of developmentally disabled individuals found that almost half felt they had benefitted from their family experiences. Another half felt they had been harmed.

Those brothers and sisters who said they had been harmed by the experience reported feeling ashamed about their retarded sibling. They reported feelings of neglect by their parents, whom they perceived as preoccupied with care of the child with special needs. These siblings blamed the child's disability for family stress. They reported childhoods overburdened with responsibility and restricted opportunities for their own recreation and growth.

In contrast, Dr. Lobato reports that those college students who said they benefitted by the situation were judged to possess many admirable personal qualities. They were described as being more compassionate and tolerant of others, as having greater understanding and sensitivity, and as being more appreciative of their own good health and intelligence than their peers. They admired their parents' dedication to their brother's or sister's special needs and felt that the disabled child had brought the family closer together.

Dr. Lobato pointed out that we should be aware of these unique concerns and intense feelings.

Siblings, especially young ones, are prone to confuse the disabled child's developmental or medical problem. Their own limitations in cognitive skills and experience get in the way. So does their parents' confusion about what information they should share, so the healthy youngster often harbors misconceptions about the cause, treatment, and potential outcome of the sibling's problem. This can result in feelings of isolation.

The healthy sibling often bears ill will toward the parents because of a perceived—or real—lack of attention. This probably plants the seeds of resentment and jealousy that some "well" siblings report feeling toward the "special-needs child." Balancing the needs of both is a key issue for parents and those who help them.

Siblings of handicapped children also report concern about the reactions of their peers to the more unusual aspects of the child's behavior or appearance. What one sibling might boast to friends as brother's or sister's accomplishment, another sibling conceals through embarrassment. Either way, most siblings are sensitive to the possibility that the attitudes and behavior of other children and adults toward them may be influenced by their sibling's status. This often influences choices of friends and eventually, spouses.

Dr. Lobato adds, "To date suggests that parental functioning, family interaction and coping styles play a major role in sibling adjustment, whereas factors such as birth order and type of disability play a more minor role."

Siblings appear to do best psychologically when their parents encourage open communication, talk about the illness or disability honestly, and don't overburden the siblings with child-care responsibilities. While open communication and information can't prevent or erase the stresses of a child's illness or disability, they are clearly important ingredients in fostering the development of understanding, compassion, and tolerance that so many siblings possess.

I am not aware of any studies focusing on the outcomes of siblings of children with ADHD specifically. In my experience, most siblings adapt well. Occasionally some embarrassment exists over their brother or sister's behavior when it is obviously out of control.

I have noted more commonly an element of jealousy growing out of the fact that the ADHD brother or sister garners a great deal more parental attention. This will occasionally lead to the healthy sibling exhibiting attention-getting behavior of his own. It also may lead to excessive teasing and "put-downs" of the ADHD child.

Parents can help counter this by making a deliberate effort to provide the non-involved sibling with appropriate acknowledgment and attention. An active ADHD child can overwhelm a parent's time and coping energy, and healthy siblings can easily, and unintentionally, be ignored.

A good move would be for parents (in a quiet moment, if they can find one) to analyze their relationships with all their children, including ones with ADHD and those with no disability. Think about ways of meeting each child's specific needs.

Try to help the healthy siblings develop some understanding of ADHD. Help them see which behaviors their brother or sister can control easily and which he or she cannot. Frequently acknowledge your appreciation for their cooperation, help, and tolerance.

For Thought and Discussion

1. Pick the life position (self-image) you think most accurately represents the self-image of your child with ADHD.

I am of value and worth.
I am not of much value or worth, but others are.
I am not of much value or worth, and neither is anyone else.
I am of value and worth, and so is everyone else.

2. What are some of the forces that influenced your child's self-image for good or bad?

3. How were you disciplined as a child? How has this affected the way you view discipline now that you are a parent?

4. Describe the temperamental characteristics of your child with ADHD. Consider factors as activity level, motivation, emotional control, and interests.

5. The following situations require encouragement. How would you respond?

   a. Your daughter complains that the math homework is too difficult.
   b. Your son has just helped you clean the kitchen.
   c. Your son is worried that he will not do well in a music recital.
   d. Your son has attempted to dress himself; his shirt is on backward, his shoes are on the wrong feet, etc.
   e. Your daughter returns from an athletic contest after playing well but having lost.

CHAPTER TEN

Strategies between Parent, Child, and School

The Place of the School in the Life of the Child

CHILDREN spend more time at school than anywhere else except home. School is not only a place where they learn the academic skills, such as the 3 R's, but it is also the place where they meet most of their friends, practice social skills, and develop many of their attitudes toward life, people, and themselves. Much of the child's sense of self-worth, or lack thereof, is determined by what happens in school.

For many children, school is the place where they experience success, achievement, and self-affirmation. We would hope this could be true for all children, but unfortunately, it is not. Many children with ADHD and other learning disabilities find school a place of failure and disappointment. It is a place where they fail—in the eyes of the school officials, their parents, and themselves. Too often, their experiences at school, rather than building up their sense of self, tear it apart.

School is more important for the child with ADHD than for most other children—in both negative and positive ways. It is often in school that their problems are first noted; at least it is when they reach school that people become concerned about their "being different." And if their problems are not identified and dealt with appropriately, school often becomes the focus of all their failure and frustration.

But the school also possesses great potential for children with ADHD. The right kind of school program can be the key in helping them work through, or get around, their problems. And most importantly, a sensitive and understanding school program can prevent many of the adverse outcomes of underachievement.

In a later chapter, we will discuss the subject of practical classroom management and teaching techniques. In this chapter, on the other hand, we seek to address the relationships between the child, parent, and school and in the process, search out ways they all can work together toward success.

Finding the Right Program for Each Child

We are not trying to present the blueprint for the perfect school. I do not know what the perfect school program looks like. In fact, I am sure there is no one perfect method or school that fits every child. In most situations, there are several alternative ways of teaching that are "right." No one method is best for every child.

The ultimate solution to the needs of the child with any disability is to individualize the teaching process. The teaching techniques used in most classrooms are the ones that over the years have been suitable for the average child. And most children usually learn adequately, if not optimally, under these conditions. But the child with ADHD or other learning disabilities may not be able to learn under these usual conditions.

Just about any child can be taught on a one-to-one basis—that is, one teacher for one child. Under such circumstances, the teacher does not have to use methods that fit the needs of many children but can respond to the unique needs of one child utilizing his own strengths and weaknesses. He can be taught the way he learns, and he can be taught at his own pace. As idealistic as this would be, such one-to-one teaching, even for the more severely impaired students, is not realistically possible in terms of personnel or finances. Yet the need to individualize is real.

Attempts to meet the individual needs of underachieving children have taken many forms. Some are more effective than others. Beginning in the 1950s, the self-contained special classroom was an honest effort at individualization. This method involved the setting up of special classes for children handicapped in any way. The purpose of such a class is to bring together children with like needs into small classes where they are taught by a trained teacher. Ideally, these classes would be small—maybe no more than eight to twelve students. At one time such classes flourished and were the primary means of giving the learning-disabled individual instruction.

But such self-contained classes do have their limitations. The children tend to be segregated from the mainstream of students and thus come to see themselves as being grossly different or odd. Too frequently, these children get "pigeon-holed" in the isolated classroom, with no attempt to bring them back into the regular class. And as the need for services to special children increased, these special education self-contained classes tended to get larger and larger until again the individual needs were lost in the crowd.

Getting in the Mainstream

In school systems across the country today, a different approach has come into use. Many names may be applied to these methods, but they are all variations of *mainstreaming*. Mainstreaming may take various forms, but in essence, it is an attempt to keep the learning-disabled child in the main flow of school activities and curriculum while still responding to his or her special needs as much as possible.

The most important tool in mainstreaming is an effective resource program. This utilizes a teacher who is trained in the latest techniques of teaching and motivation. Learning-disabled students are assigned to the resource room to get extra help for various periods during the day and spend the rest of their time in the regular classroom.

For instance, a child may be having difficulty with reading and spelling. He might spend two hours a day in a resource teacher working on reading and spelling and the rest with his peers. Jim may have difficulty in math and come only once a day for individual instruction in this subject. Billy, who is severely hyperactive, has trouble in all subjects because of his distractibility and impulsivity. He will need a more individual instruction plan. We will hear more in the near future of alternate concepts of instruction. I think we have come to see that there are no shortcuts, no magic techniques, machines, or methods. Teaching the child with ADHD or learning disabilities requires hard, innovative work. And it requires treating the child as an individual, not a square peg to be pushed into a round hold.

How Can Parents Help?

I feel that parents have a responsibility to lobby, push, yell, and scream, if necessary, to get quality programs in the schools. But then, they should leave the day-to-day teaching to those who are trained to do it. It is extremely important for parents to maintain open communication with teachers and other educators in order to know what the child's current successes and failures are and to know when new problems are developing. Success is facilitated when a cooperative partnership exists between the parent, teacher, and other professionals.

If an adequate program exists in the school, parents need not impose additional learning chores beyond the usual homework on the child at home. Such an additional academic burden only serves to frustrate the child and turn him or her away from learning entirely. We all have our breaking point. Our main job as parents is to work for proper programs in the schools, encourage both the child and his teachers, and be sensitive to related problems that may need additional attention.

What about Homework?

"I have a real fight to get my child to do his homework. What am I doing wrong?" one mother lamented.

Many parents get too involved in their children's homework. They are so uptight about their children's success that they nag and badger them until the child develops bad attitudes toward the whole learning process. We need to help our children see that learning can be fun and exciting. If such a positive attitude prevails, their school work usually will be done without a lot of pushing from us.

A parent should remember that homework is the child's responsibility—not the parent's. The parent needs to be available for assistance and counsel, but he or she should not do the homework. The parent's responsibility regarding homework is to provide the following conditions: *a place, a time, and an atmosphere* for the doing of homework. It is up to the teacher to grade the work. If the child does not do it, or does not do it well, the teacher should be the primary one to intervene.

There are times when parents and teachers will need to work closely together to set up logical consequences for the satisfactory performance of homework—or the failure to perform. By positively reinforcing an interest in learning and the good work the child does, parents can give their child the motivation to do his best without having to be pushed.

I am not saying that parents should not help the child at all. A patient, caring parent can be of practical help to the student. At times parents can assist the child by helping him organize his assignments.

The parent may, for instance, suggest that the child with ADHD do a few problems at a time and then take a break.

The parent can be available to help decipher directions, to review the work if the child asks, and to answer questions and explain confusing concepts. Certainly the parent can be interested in what the child is studying and discuss it with him. A parent involved in this manner encourages the child and reinforces the motivation to learn.

One common problem experienced by the child with ADHD is difficulty in keeping track of homework assignments. He may fail to copy the directions to begin with; leave instructions, books, etc., at school; fail to remember do the assignment even when he has the materials; or fail to hand in the homework the next day even after having done it.

Overcoming this problem is best accomplished through close cooperation between child, teacher, and parent. Some type of assignment book is needed. The teacher signs off daily, noting that the student has copied the directions correctly. The student brings the assignment book home. Parents check off when he has done the assignment.

Then it is helpful to have a special place in the workbook or backpack to place the assignments to assist the child in remembering to hand in the work in.

Medication and Homework

Children who are taking medication for their ADHD may do very well during the school day when the medication is at its optimal level, only to find homework frustrating and difficult due to a resurgence of attention and organizational problems late in the day. This pattern is common in situations where medication is taken in the morning only or morning and noon. This fall off in performance late in the day is less noticeable with the newer, long-acting forms of medication. When the child is having problems with homework, an afternoon dose may be necessary. Also, if this problem exists, it may be helpful for the student to do the homework early in the afternoon rather than waiting until late in the evening.

The Importance of Parent-Teacher Communication

Regardless of the kind of educational setting your child is in, communication between you and the teacher is vital. For all practical purposes, you are the coordinator of services for your child. You need to know what is happening to, and with, your child on a regular, frequent basis.

Too often parents become aware of delinquent work, changed work habits, or difficult behavior only after these have reached crisis proportions. At this point, the child and the teacher are frustrated. It would be much better to anticipate such problems in the early stages and institute preventative strategies before the crisis develops. This can only be done if parent and teacher stay in close communication.

Second, parents need to be in a position to acknowledge and reinforce (reward) progress as it occurs (hopefully each small step toward progress). As discussed in the chapter on discipline, both punishments and rewards are much more effective if immediate and given in small, incremental steps. If parents really want to motivate their child to try as hard as he or she can, they must reward effort and improved performance on a frequent, even daily, basis. On the other hand, parents should not try to become part of the classroom or bug the teacher constantly with their own ideas and questions.

The proper approach is something like this. The parent can say to the teacher:

> I appreciate all that you are doing for Jim (or Betty, etc.).
> I am concerned that he do the best he can and that he
> have the benefit of all the school can provide. I would

like to keep in touch with you on a regular basis in case I can do something to reinforce what you are doing in the classroom. Could we have a conference often until we see how he is doing? Also, would you let me know immediately if a problem develops?

At other times, particularly at the start of therapy or a new remedial program, there is a need to have daily communication between parent and teacher. An assignment notebook can be sent back and forth. Daily contact via the telephone may be helpful. Today, more and more parents and teachers are finding that e-mail is an efficient way to stay in touch.

If the parents take an affirming, cooperative approach with the teacher(s), the teacher most likely will be open and cooperative. Parents should avoid a demanding, accusatory attitude. It is important for parents to remember that their child and teacher must work together for at least a year. They should try not to strain that relationship. If parents have a disagreement with the teacher, they should not discuss this with the child. Neither should they criticize the teacher in front of the child. If there is a problem, the parent may need to speak to the teacher in private. When the child becomes a pawn between a combative teacher and parent, the child is the big loser.

Public vs. Private School

Which is best? Should my child be in public or private school? Is there a special school for learning-disabled kids?

There are no simple answers to these questions. In some communities, private schools exist that are flexible enough to meet the individual needs of the learning-disabled child. But many private schools cater only to the high achievers and have little patience for the child with any kind of learning difference.

At the same time, in more and more communities, public schools are expanding their programs to offer a wide range of diagnostic and remedial services to all handicapped children. Most of the time public schools will have more resources to offer than typical private school.

However, there are many competing needs in public schools, and large class size may be a problem.

The rare community will have a private schools designed especially for learning- disabled children. Unfortunately, such programs are usually very expensive, and few parents can afford them. Some smaller private schools may, through their flexibility and small classes, be suitable placements for the child with ADHD or a learning disability.

The question of public vs. private school must be answered conditionally, taking into account the unique needs of the child and the resources of the community.

What about Tutoring?

Tutoring is probably the oldest method of providing help to the underachieving child. A recent study evaluating the success of young adults who were learning-disabled as children showed that those who had effective tutoring did better than the average. To be effective, tutoring must be carried out correctly. The tutoring teacher must be competent, and the program must be tailored to the child. However, parents should not expect too much from one hour a day of tutoring when the child is faced with frustration and underachievement six to eight hours a day in school.

Tutoring cannot take the place of a proper school program, and if such a program exists, then tutoring may not be necessary. However, a sensitive, well-designed tutoring program may at times be a worthwhile adjunct to the overall teaching program. Tutoring may be of particular value in helping a child catch up in one isolated subject in which he is deficient. Sometimes it can help a struggling learning-disabled child maintain his academic gains during the summer.

However, I would caution against piling time-consuming tutoring sessions into a child's already busy day. A child who has had a full day at school doesn't have much emotional energy left to cope with an hour of tutoring after school. The child with problems needs time to be a child—to run free, to daydream, to do nothing. We need to remember that simply piling on more hours of academic study will not solve a child's academic problem and indeed, is likely to increase frustration, which, in turn, decreases efficiency.

A Final Note

The parent, child, and teacher are a team. The more closely they work together, communicate, and have common goals, the more likely they will be to experience success. And success for one is success for all.

For Thought and Discussion

1. List all the people in your child's school with whom you should communicate.

2. What are some things you can do as a parent to improve communication with school personnel?

CHAPTER ELEVEN

Success Unlimited: the Future

Encouraging News

IN chapter 1, we considered the five questions that trouble parents of struggling children. So far in this book we have tried to touch base with all of these questions and provide the best answers our knowledge now permits.

The last of the five questions is the one that provokes the most anxiety: *"What is the future of my child?"*

This stirs still more questions:

"Will he finish school?"
"Will she go to college?"
"Will he get a job?"
"What kind of person will she be when she grows up?"

Until recently, more confusion than answers have surrounded these questions. Some children made it, and some didn't. Some with ADHD became more and more alienated from peers and society and experienced chronic failure; others seemed to settle down, becoming successful students. But there was little data with which to make accurate predictions about individual children. In the last few years, however, researchers have pieced together a more coherent picture of the future of children with ADHD.

A few years ago, several workers from McGill University in Canada published in *The Archives of General Psychiatry6* a follow-up study of sixty-four children with ADHD. Although these children received some medical and educational therapy, it was sporadic and of a short duration. At the time of this study, most of the children were teenagers. Obvious hyperactivity had indeed lessened. Disorders of attention and concentration had improved but were present in many. A significant number of the children were underachievers as teens and suffered poor self-concepts. Some had serious emotional problems.

Of particular importance is that most of these children received less than optimal educational, behavioral, and medical therapy. In general, this study provided us with a picture of what happens to the untreated or partially treated child with ADHD. It showed that, indeed, many of the neuro-developmental symptoms could persist into adolescence and adulthood.

N. W. Laufer reported in the *Journal of Learning Disabilities7* the results of a follow-up study of sixty comprehensively treated children with hyperactivity. Their treatment included appropriate medication, counseling, and educational therapy. The average age at which treatment began was eight years, and the average time of follow-up was twenty years. In 23 percent of the children, medication was used for five years or more. Of the forty-eight children for which complete data were available, 29 percent were in college or had received a degree. Some were attending graduate school. Forty-seven percent were in high school or had graduated. Thus, 76 percent had received, or were receiving, a higher education. Only 5 percent were deferred for lack of fitness for military service due to emotional reasons. Excessive alcohol intake was a problem in 8 percent of those studied. Five percent had a history of drug abuse of some kind (about average for the general population).

Dr. Lily Hecktman and Bagrielle Weis published a study of individuals with ADHD who were young adults at the time of the study. They noted that most of these young adults who had been hyperactive as children were basically well adjusted. Only ten out of the seventy-six studied had any significant adjustment or emotional problems. The most common deficiencies noted were in self-esteem and social skills.

---

6   Weiss, G., *Arch. Gen. Psychiatry.*, 24:409–414, May 1971 .
7   Laufer, M., J., *Learning Disabilities*, 4:55–58.

(The negative feedback children with ADHD experienced throughout the developing years leaves a definite mark on their self-esteem.)

Dr. James Shatterfield and colleagues[8] reported the results of their study of one hundred boys with ADHD who received combined therapy including educational help, counseling, and medication as needed. Those receiving the most help were the most advanced educationally, had less antisocial behavior, were more attentive, and were better adjusted than those receiving no treatment.

Although until recently more confusion than answers have surrounded these questions, four significant conclusions can be drawn from these and similar studies.

1. These results are compatible with what most of us working with ADHD have observed over the years. *Children who are properly treated have a wide range of occupational possibilities and can, and do, achieve, learn, grow, and mature.* Most come to adulthood with a sound self-image in spite of the problems they have had to overcome. Their hyperactivity does abate somewhat, and they develop better organization and work habits. They find ways to compensate for many of their weaknesses. Large numbers of such children have gone on to achieve in fields as diverse as engineering, teaching, business, and medicine.

I was recently the advisor to a medical student who as a child had ADHD and a severe learning disability. Yet she had been able to graduate from a prestigious university and work her way to the senior year of medical school.

2. These studies illustrate the importance of early comprehensive treatment. Without intervention, the child is vulnerable to failure, emotional disturbance, and personal disappointment.

3. These same studies point out that although children with ADHD tend to have a natural attenuation of their symptoms as they move into adolescence, some characteristics of ADHD tend to persist even into adulthood. The milder a child's symptoms, the more likely he will be relatively free of symptoms as a teenager. The more severely involved child is more likely to have persisting symptoms.

Symptoms in adolescents are likely to be more subtle. Involved adolescents tend to have difficulty attending, organizing, and putting things in order. Coordination often improves significantly at puberty,

---

8   Satterfield, J., *Amer. Acad. Child Adol. Psychiatry.*, 26:56–64.

but perceptual problems may not improve much. In fact, the teen with ADHD may easily be missed. Unfortunately, the teen with attention and organizational problems is in danger of being labeled as lazy or unmotivated Untreated, they can become discouraged, experience increasing cycles of failure, and eventually just give up.

4. In some individuals, symptoms of attention deficit persist into adulthood. In fact, physicians are now realizing that certain adults have significant problems with concentration, organization, and sequencing and will benefit from medication.

The Ultimate Goal

Remember our ultimate goal for all children, whatever their assets, is that they grow into responsible and responsive adults who know their strengths and limitations but who have the self-confidence to make the most of their unique personality and gifts.

I strongly believe this kind of success is possible with every child. In this workbook, we have outlined the strategy for accomplishing this. Success comes from a cooperative effort on the part of parents, child, professionals, and school personnel. So with an air of optimism, let us all pull together for *success.*

For Thought and Discussion

1. List five personal strengths of your child that could help him or her succeed in life:

2. What are some hurdles your child will need to overcome in order to succeed?

3. What are some things you can do to help your child maximize his or her strengths and overcome his or her weaknesses?

SECTION FOUR
MORE STRATEGIES

CHAPTER TWELVE

The Spectrum of Specific Learning Disabilities

Do You Know This Boy?

Percy F., a well-groomed lad, age fourteen, is the eldest son of intelligent parents, the second in a family of seven. He always has been a bright and intelligent boy, quick at games, and in no way inferior to others of his age. His greatest difficulty—his inability to learn to read—is remarkable and pronounced. He has been at school or under tutors since he was seven years old, and with the greatest of this laborious and persistent training, he can only with difficulty spell words of one syllable. The schoolmaster who has taught him for some years says that he would be the smartest lad in the school if the instructions were entirely oral.

Many reading this book will recognize Percy. I dare say every elementary classroom teacher has seen him at one time or another. They may know him as Billy, Sue, Betty, or Danny, but, whatever their names, the Percys of this world present a dilemma: they have all the appearances of bright, alert, well-adjusted children, but they meet with failure and frustration in one or more of the common academic tasks, such as reading, spelling, writing, and calculating.

This description of Percy was provided in 1896 by a British physician,

W. Pringle Morgan, writing in the *British Journal of Medicine.9* Dr. Morgan's perceptive report is one of the first descriptions of a learning-disabled child to appear in scientific literature. Dr. Morgan was a model for us—for he saw young *Percy not as a problem child but as a child with a problem.*

Since 1896, many additional facts have been uncovered about such children who have difficulty in learning:

The most common academic problem is that of learning to read.

- Learning and reading problems are more common in boys than in girls.
- Such problems often run in families.
- Many successful people have suffered with learning disabilities as children but have overcome them with a great deal of effort.
- But many children, overwhelmed with frustration and failure, give up, drop out of academic efforts, and become emotional and behavioral underachievers due to the frustration.

Defining Learning Disabilities

Beginning in the 1930s and 1940s, research into learning disabilities by the educational, psychological, and medical disciplines intensified. Many people attempted to define causative factors and remedial techniques. One of the earliest labels to be used to define such children as described by Dr. Morgan was "dyslexia," which literally means, "inability to recognize words."

Physicians, educators, and psychologists have had difficulty over the years defining dyslexia. It means different things to different people but often is used as a general term to define a child, such as Percy F., who is bright but can't learn efficiently in the same manner as other children.

In the 1950s and 1960s, the term Minimal Brain Injury (MBI) or Minimal Brain Damage (MBD) came into use as a result of the belief that most learning disabilities were due to anatomic damage to the brain. Later, these terms were discarded in favor of Minimal

—————————————————

9   Morgan, P, "A case of congenital word blindness," *British Journal of Medicine,* 2:1378, 1896.

Brain Dysfunction. It was felt to be more accurate because no apparent brain injury could be found in most children with learning problems. The rationale behind this thinking was that learning-disabled children presented many of the characteristics of children and adults with known brain damage, even though proof of brain damage was lacking in most children.

In the later 1960s, a general consensus developed that terms such as Minimal Brain Damage and Minimal Brain Dysfunction were inadequate and too emotionally charged to label most poor learners, so most professionals moved toward a more functional classification, which finally led to the term *Specific Learning Disability*. This term was incorporated into federal legislation and has persisted in the language of most specialists.

Definition

The Council for Exceptional Children met in St. Louis in April of 1967 and prepared the following definition of learning disabilities:

> A child with learning disabilities is one with adequate mental abilities, sensory processes, and emotional stability, who has a limited number of specific deficits in perceptive, integrative, or expressive processes which severely impair learning efficiency. This includes children who have a central nervous system dysfunction, which is expressed primarily in impaired learning efficiency.

The National Advisory Committee on Handicapped Children in January of 1968 expanded somewhat their definition as follows:

> Children with specific learning disabilities exhibit a disorder in one or more of the basic psychological processes involved in understanding or in using spoken or written languages. These may be manifested in disorders of listening, thinking, talking, reading, writing, spelling, or arithmetic. They include conditions which have been referred to as perceptual handicaps, brain injury, minimal

brain dysfunction, dyslexia, developmental aphasia, and so on. They do not include learning problems which are due primarily to visual, hearing, or motor handicaps, to mental retardation, emotional disturbance, or environmental disadvantages.

It is this definition that was incorporated into the landmark federal legislation of 1975 concerning education of the handicapped (PL 94: 142, 1975).

You may still see the term dyslexia used by some professionals. Most people use dyslexia interchangeably with learning disabilities. More specifically, however, dyslexia as a diagnosis implies a constitutional, neurological basis for reading difficulties.

Other Conditions Affecting Learning

Children may underachieve in school for many reasons besides actual learning disabilities. Let us look at some of these before we proceed with our discussion of specific learning disabilities.

1. *Physical Handicaps.*

Physical handicaps, such as hearing loss, visual problems, and muscle or skeletal problems, can interfere with a child's ability to respond in the classroom, thus adversely affecting his performance.

2. *Lack of Opportunity.*

A child who has not previously been exposed to a learning environment or been encouraged to learn may be behind academically. This may be noticeable in kindergarten or first grade when the child has not been exposed to learning before. Such a child can learn. He simply has not yet developed the tools for learning.

3. *Poor Learning Environment.*

Some academic environments simply are not conducive to learning. A personality conflict may exist between the teacher and child. They cannot work as a team and the child does not learn.

Another example of a poor learning environment contributing to a child's underachievement is when the child moves from an inferior school to a better one. Suddenly his grades plummet because he is behind the pace of his new school. When faced with this situation, most students will catch up within a short time if given some reasonable help.

4. *Stress.*

A child who is under significant or continuous stress may have deteriorating grades. Stress, if severe or prolonged, decreases one's mental alertness and efficiency. With acute stress (such as from family problems, sickness, a move), there may be sudden deterioration in the academic work level. Usually there will be other observable symptoms of stress in the child's life.

5. *Lower Mental Abilities*

A child in whom the overall ability level is well below his or her age level will have difficultly learning at a normal pace. Because of this overall decrease in ability, learning will be impaired. The mentally retarded child will require appropriate teaching on his or her mental age level.

Characteristics of Learning Disability

To understand what happens with the learning-disabled child, it would help to review the steps in the learning process.

In order for learning to take place, there must be a *stimulus*—that is, there must be information to be learned (for instance, the alphabet, a series of words, geometry theory, etc.). Once there is a stimulus, the pupil must *attend to* (pay attention to) the stimulus for a sufficient length of time for it to be fixed in the mind. We are surrounded all the time by a variety of stimuli we do not remember (or learn) because they never catch our attention. Once we have attended to the information, our sense organs must *register, or sense,* the information and transmit it via nerves to the brain, where it *is processed.*

Of course, for one to learn to read a series of words, it is necessary for the brain to *perceive* accurately the words themselves (i.e., it is necessary for the brain to see the words as they actually are with the proper shape and orientation, not upside down or twisted out of shape).

Once the information is perceived, a complex *processing* of the information occurs. In reading, for instance, auditory and visual signals must be properly associated and integrated in the brain. Then the information is *recorded in the short-term memory.* This means one has immediate recall of what he has just perceived. For instance, if a child looks at the letters of the alphabet and then turns and immediately writes them down, he is using his short-term memory.

It is possible for one to be able to write the letters immediately after seeing them but not be able to do it the next day. That is because the information has not been recorded in the long-term memory. Only as the information *is firmly fixed in the long-term memory* is it really learned. For this cycle of learning to be complete, the student must be able to *retrieve* the information from the memory when needed and *express* it in some meaningful way.

Blocks in this stream of learning can occur anywhere along this pathway. Initially, the child must attend the stimulus to be learned long enough to latch onto it. Failure to adequately concentrate on the information to be learned results in inefficient, inconsistent learning. The child with an attention deficit (as mentioned earlier) has trouble precisely at this point.

In specific learning disabilities, the processing of information by the central nervous system is disrupted somewhere in the order of these complex operations. This may involve an alteration in the perception, organization, storage, retrieval, or expression of information to be learned. To summarize, leaning goes through these steps:

- Perception (hearing, seeing, feeling)
- Integration
- Memory
- Expression (written, oral, action)

This brief description of this intricate process is provided to illustrate the many points at which learning can be disrupted. The evaluation of learning difficulties of a specific child requires careful observation and often testing by an experienced diagnostician.

Summary

This short, somewhat superficial, overview of the learning process is not intended to be exhaustive. Rather, it seeks to give parents and teachers insight into how learning occurs and how it may be blocked. An underachieving child may have a limited defect in only one of these areas. Others may have a more pervasive disability, with problems in several of these functions. If anything, I am impressed with the fact that no two learning-disabled children are alike.

Many children with deficiencies in one or more of these functions also may have attention deficit disorders with or without hyperactivity. Of course, when we have this kind of combination, the child's practical problems are compounded. For a child who is underachieving educationally, psychologically, and neurologically, testing will be helpful in defining the nature and degree of their dysfunction so treatment may be planned.

A Special Note to Teachers

In another chapter, I make some general suggestions for working with the learning-disabled child in the classroom. However, in that chapter or elsewhere in this book, I do not attempt to tell teachers how to teach. Education is a complex profession in itself, and competent educators have a wide repertoire of teaching methods. In this book, I simply try to help parents, educators, and others appreciate the uniqueness of learning-disabled children and to understand the neuro-developmental basis for their difficulties.

For Thought and Discussion

1. Have you or your child's teacher had any concerns your child's overall school performance? Which area?

2. Does your child show signs of any of the learning dysfunctions discussed in this chapter?

3. List the resource people in your school you can talk to about your child's learning progress:

CHAPTER THIRTEEN

"I've Always Wondered Why"

The Need to Know Why

"Why can't Judy learn to read?"
"Why is Sammy's behavior so difficult to control?"
"Why is Bobby hyperactive?"
"Why?"

This is one of the most persistent questions I hear from parents. This is true when Sandy has only a cold or an ear infection. It is even more pervasive when it is a problem as complicated and involved as a behavior disorder or learning disability. "Why" is a valid question that needs a response as we move on to management or treatment of any developmental condition. Actually, both parents and professionals have a deep, underlying need to know why.

But of course, other important reasons exists for knowing the why, or cause, of a condition like attention deficit or learning disability. Most importantly, if we know the ultimate cause, we can be more specific in our prevention and treatment.

The Search for an Answer

"Why?" has proven to be a most difficult question to answer when it comes to ADHD. When it comes to the inner workings of the brain, we just do not know enough. Even though great strides have been made, it seems we know less about the human brain and how it functions than we do about the surface of the moon or the atmosphere of Venus. The brain has been mapped, its cells studied under microscope, and its chemical contents analyzed. But how an organ that looks so simple can perform all the functions the brain does is just beyond our understanding.

The mechanical tasks, such as sensory awareness, number calculation, and muscle control, are themselves incomprehensible enough. But when we consider memory, concept formation, perception, and creativity, it is a marvel that the brain functions as well as it does. Since we do not understand normal function, we certainly have difficulty understanding why the brain does not always work the same in all people. Current research using new, high-powered tools is pushing back the curtain of ignorance with warp speed. Wide gaps still exist in our knowledge about how we learn, acquire information, process it, store it, and use it, but every day we are learning something new about this process. New information is helping us understand more and more about the underlying anatomical and chemical variations associated with ADHD.

However, until this curtain of ignorance is pushed back further, we cannot be too dogmatic about the causes of conditions such as ADHD and learning disabilities.

In order to better understand the present state of scientific research into hyperactivity, attention deficit, learning disabilities, and related problems, we need to review some history. Over the years, various theories about the cause have come and gone. These have varied from different concepts of brain injury to simple environmental causes. Others have claimed that there was no such thing as a hyperactive child—only personality conflicts between the child and certain adults. The hyperactivity and related problems are claimed to be "in the eyes of the beholder."

Fortunately, we now have more concrete, if not complete, data by which to judge the issue. In the last three decades, the research has focused less on brain injury and more on the biochemical function of the brain. A variety of scientific studies now suggests that the balance of various chemicals and hormones present in very small amounts are an integral part of brain function. Further research has shown that certain abnormalities in these brain biochemicals do affect nervous system function and behavior.

More recently, the study of brain function has become an exciting area of research. Preliminary studies suggest subtle differences between ADHD and other children. The data so far from a variety of studies suggest small but significant variations in how the brain works in hyperactive children.

Back to Why!

Some parents may be interested in this discussion of history and chemistry. Some clearly are not. But the question in the mind of just about every parent I have met is, "Why?"

"Why this chemical imbalance or whatever?"

"Why this neuro-developmental disorganization? Why this hyperactivity?"

These are legitimate questions, but they are ones that are not always easily answered. Let's look at some of the possible causes of hyperactivity that have been proposed over the years!

1. *Heredity*

Some interesting circumstantial evidence exists to suggest genetics play a significant role in predisposing one to experience ADHD. For a long time it has been known that both ADHD and many learning disorders are more common in males, suggesting genetic factors. Those working with such children are struck by the frequency of a father or mother saying, "I was just like that myself when I was a child. I almost didn't finish school." It is not uncommon to have two or more siblings in the family with varying degrees of ADHD. More recent research suggests that genetic factors play a most important part in predisposing one to attention deficits.

2. *Structural Brain Injury*

As far back as 1934, Dr. Al Kahn presented a paper in *The New England Journal of Medicine* in which he discussed a syndrome seen in patients who had recovered from encephalitis. Hyperactivity, inability to concentrate, clumsiness, and emotional explosiveness were common to all of these patients. Dr. Kahn spoke of these patients as being "driven" by internal forces beyond their control: "The patient seems to be a puppet at the mercy of his malfunctioning brain stem," he reported.[10]

The consequences of birth trauma and other forms of central nervous system injury were studied extensively in the 1950s and 1960s. By far, prematurity is the most common obstetric complication associated with mental and physical handicaps of all kinds, including learning and behavior problems. In a study of five hundred infants, Dr. Hilda Knoblach and Benjamin Pasamanick documented the relationship of prematurity to handicaps such as cerebral palsy, seizures, mental deficits, and behavioral and learning problems. They also found that the more premature the infant, the more likely the child is to have a handicap.

No doubt prenatal and postnatal problems account for a few children with ADHD or learning disabilities. The majority of children do not have any evidence of such specific brain injury in their medical history.

3. *Allergy and toxic reactions*

Many parents and teachers have heard of various theories about food hypersensitivity and other allergies causing hyperactivity, attention problems, and learning disabilities. Various authors have suggested that a large number of children can be cured through adherence to a defined diet that restricts a variety of foods and food additives. Independent research carried out by many investigators has not duplicated the positive results reported by most of these proponents.

The evidence from many well-controlled studies shows that food allergies do not play a major role in causing attention and activity problems. Based on these studies as well as clinical observations, it is now clear that allergy to foods or other ingested substances (such as additives) is rarely, if ever, a *primary* cause of hyperactivity and learning dysfunction.

However, for a few children, intolerance or allergy to certain substances may aggravate, or worsen, the expression of their symptoms. I have noted in my own practice an occasional patient whose behavior and performance improved modestly when certain substances are restricted from the diet.

---

10   Kahn, A, Organic Driveness, NEJM, 210:248-256

Pediatricians know that certain medicines will cause hyperactivity and impulsiveness in certain children. For instance, medicines used to treat asthma will cause the patient to become more active and less controlled. Phenobarbital and other barbiturates used to treat seizures will also cause this reaction. When such medicines are used with children who have ADHD, more acting out and aggressive behavior can be expected.

In my own practice, I will consider investigating dietary factors, or other allergens, when there is a strong history of allergy in the child (and his family) and when parents, from their own observations, suspect an association between the ingestion of certain foods and behavior. One father had noted that his seven-year-old son seemed to become much more hyperactive after visiting their favorite Mexican food restaurant. Finally it dawned on him that his son gulped dozens of red-colored taco chips. Following this hint, we determined that, indeed, this child had hypersensitivity to a red dye. Knowing this, the parents could restrict this one product, but there was no need for a broad-spectrum diet restriction.

Standard allergy testing is of little help. The only way to adequately assess such food allergies is by means of an elimination diet. This involves taking the child off all foods containing the suspected villain for two weeks. Then gradually, the suspect food is added back into the diet. Behavior is observed closely with and without the suspected food in the diet. Although somewhat complicated, this procedure can help identify offending dietary factors when they do exist.

There are problems with the highly restrictive diet as proposed by some that remove many common foods. Such a limited diet disrupts the family routine and can lead to conflict between the child and parents. It can also lead to some nutritional deficiencies if not monitored closely. When necessary, a modified elimination diet can be used. In this, only suspected foods or substances are eliminated for the trial period. I encourage you to consult your physician before attempting such a diet.

4. *Refined Sugar*

Over the years, parents at times have reported that the behavior of their child seems to worsen after the child has ingested a sugar.

In the last several years, many studies have looked at the effect of sugar on behavior. Most of these have shown sugar intake to have little overall effect on behavior. A study performed in 1986 by Dr. Jane Goldman and her associates at the University of Connecticut looked at this issue from a little different perspective.

They evaluated behavior at different times following sugar ingestion. They found that behavior did get worse forty-five to sixty minutes after a large sugar snack. This period of worsening behavior lasted an hour or two, after which behavior returned to its normal state. Another study suggested that a high-carbohydrate diet made an individual more susceptible to the effects of sugar. We can hope that ongoing research in the near future will shed more light on this.

I frequently recommend a low to moderate sugar intake for children with ADHD whom I treat. It may help them, and it certainly cannot hurt. There is no doubt that we Americans, children and adults, eat too much refined sugar, to the detriment of our general health. If nothing else, such high sugar intake encourages dental cavities, causes obesity, and may decrease our desire for other, more nutritious foods.

5. *Stress*

Since the syndrome of ADHD was first described, some professionals have denied its neurological basis, proclaiming it was simply another emotional adjustment disorder. In their thinking, attention deficit, impulsivity, and hyperactivity are simply the result of stress and maladjustment in the child's life. According to this theory, dysfunctions do not originate within the child but in the child's environment. If only the stress was removed, then the child's symptoms would clear up.

Adequate evidence exists to thoroughly refute this concept. No child developmental issue has been studied more than that of ADHD and related neurological disorders. From working with hundreds of such children, I know that they come from all kinds of family backgrounds.

Certainly, some children come from environments that are not ideal, environments where there is a lack of nurturing and where stress and pressure are excessive. But most children come from average, normal families, and most parents of hyperactive and children with ADHD are rearing other children successfully. I know that hyperactivity and learning disability are not caused simply by emotional maladjustment or bad parenting.

However, there is no doubt that stress of any kind tends to aggravate all the definitive symptoms of ADHD and learning disability, making adjustment and success much more difficult for the child. Such stress can come in many forms. Discord in the parents' marriage, undue pressure on the child to meet unrealistic goals, family financial difficulties, or a depressed or disturbed parent can, and will, aggravate the underlying expression of ADHD.

If there is this kind of stress in the child's life, it will rarely go away on its own. The parents, the child, or the family as a whole will need some professional counseling. Such counseling may be obtained from a variety of professionals: physicians, psychologists, school counselors, social workers, pastors, etc. A support group of parents with common needs can be a major help in dealing with the pressures and stresses in their own life and in their relationships with their children.

If undue stresses exist in your family and in your relationship with your child, seek help. Talk to your physician, your pastor, or a specialist at a community guidance center. All the other treatment measures will be of limited success until attention is given to these family stresses and pressures.

Any of these aggravating factors may, or may not, play a significant part in your child's problems. When they are suspected, remedial measures can be undertaken to deal with them. Once this is done, you then can look at the other necessary steps in the overall management strategy.

Let's Keep an Open Mind

Today we know that the predisposition to ADHD is inherited. At times there may be other factors contributing to the expression of the symptoms.

If I can clearly identify the cause of hyperactivity, attention deficit, or learning disability in a child, I am glad to share this with the parents. When I can't, I am honest with them.

Someday we may be able to identify the causative factors better than we now can. I suspect that we will find that the cause of hyperactivity and attention deficit is multi-factorial—that is, many factors interact to produce the syndrome. For instance, there may be a genetic predisposition, which is then activated by such stresses as brain injury, infection, or other yet to be identified factors. Hopefully, current research will continue to illuminate our ignorance at this point.

We Know What Did Not Cause It!

My experience as a parent and as a pediatrician has taught me much about parental guilt. As mentioned in previous chapters, I have decided that guilt is one of the most common and natural of parental emotions.

When something happens to one of our children, our automatic response is to blame ourselves. Our brain computer searches its memory bank until it comes up with some trivial event, which we then focus on as the cause. Thus, we feel guilty. We just know that our child is all messed up because of something we didn't do that we should have or because we did something we should not have done. I see this daily in my office. I spend much of my time trying to convince parents that their children's illness is not their fault.

As discussed earlier, this parental guilt reaction is even more intense when the child has a behavior or learning problem. Again, with these conditions the primary cause is almost never the fault of the parents. This is particularly true of parents of children with hyperactivity and learning disabilities. These children are driven by an internal motor that is not dependent on external fuel. Some "experts" would attribute hyperactive behavior and related symptoms solely to inappropriate actions of the parents. But more often than not, it is the other way around: the child's abnormal, disruptive behavior is itself a cause of parental tension and frustration.

Let's Move on to More Important Things

It is natural for both parents and professionals to think in terms of cause. And certainly, when possible, the cause should be identified. But it is detrimental to the welfare of the child for parents and professionals to become so preoccupied with diagnosis of causative factors that they never get around to proper treatment. Surely treatment is the most important part of our strategy for success. And regardless of the cause, the treatment of hyperactivity, attention deficit, and learning disabilities follow some basic patterns. The rest of this book is dedicated to practical, strategies that will help the child, the family, and his school work toward ultimate success and application.

For Thought and Discussion

1. Are you still asking yourself "why?"?

2. What things or events have you considered as a possible cause of your child's symptoms?

3. Have you had your questions answered to your satisfaction?

4. How much have you been affected by guilt over your child's condition?

CHAPTER FOURTEEN

*Classroom Strategies—Teaching
the Hard to Teach Child*

The Teacher's Challenge

I have great admiration for the dedicated teacher, and most teachers I know are teaching because they love children and like being around them. They have a sense of satisfaction when they see their students learn, grow, and succeed.

On the other hand, they are frustrated and personally defeated when one of their students fails to achieve and succeed. Thus the presence of a learning-disabled or hyperactive student in a class tends to stir up a mixture of reactions in a conscientious teacher. He or she wants to help but is thwarted by lack of time, too many students, or a lack of materials or training. This easily leads to frustration and hopelessness.

One fourth-grade teacher spoke not only for herself, but also many colleagues, when she discussed a learning-disabled child in her class. "Jimmy is a puzzle. I want to help him, but I've been frustrated at every turn."

This section cannot offer solutions to all the problems involved in teaching the learning-disabled child. The information presented here is a potpourri of tried and proven techniques that have been gleaned from experienced teachers. Hopefully, they will make the job of teaching the child with ADHD or learning disabilities a little less frustrating and more rewarding for you and the children in your class.

A Quick Review ADHD

Up to this point, we have learned many things about children with attention deficit. We have learned that they have three major areas of dysfunction:

- Disordered attention control
- Disordered impulse control
- Disordered activity control

These behaviors result in a mixed bag of behaviors that, to a greater or lesser degree, affects the child's ability to adjust, learn, and relate. Some of these behaviors are:

1. Short attention span
2. Distractibility
3. Slowed reaction time
4. Delayed motor speed
5. Poor response to reinforcements (to discipline)
6. Rapid mood changes with poor control of emotional expression
7. Poor self-monitoring
8. Inability to stop, look, and listen before acting
9. Inefficiency in sequencing, patterning, and organizing their world

These behavioral and learning differences result from neuro-developmental dysfunction due to physical and developmental problems. (See chapter 3 for more details.) We also have learned that all children with ADD and ADHD are not the same. All do not have the same behavior repertoire. The eventual behavior the child exhibits at home, in the classroom, and on the playground is a product of several forces that combine to mold the child's behavior.

Thus, children with attention deficit disorder come in a variety of packages. Some have minimal hyperactivity, attention deficits, and impulsiveness; their daily life is not noticeably affected except at times and points of demand and stress. Others are more totally involved and have problems of adjustment at every turn; success in most all things eludes them.

Classroom Strategies

From long experience, we know that children with hyperactivity and attention deficits function much better in an organized, structured atmosphere. Not only does such an atmosphere allow the child to function more efficiently in the present, but it also encourages him to internalize this imposed organization so that, in time, the child becomes more self-controlled.

The following suggestions regarding classroom management have been derived from the available literature, current research findings, and clinical observations. The goal of these strategies is to help the child internalize control of attention, impulsiveness, and activity, thus improving work habits and general behavior. The methods are designed to help the child develop more conscious control. Each teacher will not, and should not, employ each and every technique presented. This is simply a sampling of practical techniques that can help with certain problem behaviors. The teacher can pick those he or she thinks may work for him or her with the child in question.

Classroom Strategies Useful with ADHD Children

1) Seat the student near the teacher's desk in a reassuring, nonthreatening way.
2) Call the student's name before addressing him or asking him to recite.
3) Stand near the child when giving instructions.
4) Since the physical features of the work environment influence the activity and distractibility level, consider the following:
   - Reduce the visual stimuli in the child's visual field (place construction paper over windows, eliminate posters, pictures, etc.)
   - Lighting should be of medium intensity, with no flickering or bright lights.

- Try to schedule work so the child is not being expected to concentrate when there is a lot of distracting noise in the hallway.
- Music set at a low volume can be helpful in masking continuous distractions.
- For children with significant attention deficits, create a private study office by screening off an area for work.

5) A child with ADHD will often have difficulty finishing work. Give shorter assignments with immediate feedback of results. Multiple short assignments work better than one long assignment.

6) Work from small units to larger units in the quantity of work required, the complexity of the task, and time required to complete tasks.

- Shorten assignments.
- Start with easily accomplished tasks.
- Build assignments in terms of length and complexity.
- Plan interruptions of long assignments.
- Cut worksheets (e.g., arithmetic) into long strips, and present each strip individually.
- Vary activity.
- Use techniques, such as assignment cards, that help improve short-term memory.
- List each activity.
- If necessary, list steps in a specific activity.
- Indicate approximate time limits to be spent on major activities.
- Use check marks when assignments are completed (or steps are completed).
- Tape card to desk or tote tray.
- Use unique, distinct visual and auditory stimuli by underlining, color coding, and/or specific verbal direction.
- Cue the child to distinguish features of each stimulus in reading or arithmetic.
- Provide an opportunity to express motor restlessness in appropriate ways.

Summary

As I said earlier, there are no easy answers to treating and teaching children with attention deficits. These children are often lovable and attractive, while at the same time frustrating and exhausting to the teacher. One or two such children in a regular classroom without help for the teacher can be stressful for everyone. Open, free communication between teacher, parent, physician, and educational diagnostician is of critical importance if success is to be realized.

While the institution of a well-structured, organized environment at home and school will allow many hyperactive children to function reasonably well, others will need additional modes of therapy, such as medication or a prescribed behavior modification plan. However, the teacher is always a key member of the management team.

Classroom Strategies Useful with Learning-Disabled Children

There is no one magic technique—no easy solutions for teaching the learning-disabled child. Each one needs to be approached as an individual. The learning-disabled child is like a lock that is rusted and tightly shut. The teacher has a handful of keys but doesn't know which one works. The teacher and his or her consultants must try the ring of keys until they find one that unlocks the mystery of the individual child's learning processes. Listed below are a few keys gleaned from many experienced teachers.

Specific Teaching Procedures and Classroom Modifications

It would be futile to attempt to list a specific set of procedures that would be appropriate for all learning-disabled children, since the symptoms of each student differ from those of others. There are, however, some specific teaching procedures, classroom modifications, and attitudes that will increase your chance of success as a teacher. Some of these specific procedures and modifications follow:

1) Foster an atmosphere that accepts individual differences.

Those working with the learning-disabled child need to see him/her as a child with a problem, not a problem child. The child needs help, not condemnation.

- Be patient and optimistic. Each child has his own rate of learning, as well as his time table for physical and social development.
- Look for each child's strengths, and encourage and reinforce these islands of potential and achievement. The poor reader may have strength in math, music, or oral communication. Each has a gift.

2) Permit the child to use learning aids as long as needed without penalty

- Some children need a reading window (slot in a card) to keep them from losing their place.
- Allow use of fingers or other concrete materials for counting when working math problems.
- Carrying and borrowing marks will help the child focus and remember.
- Allow the child to print if this is easier for him. For some learning-disabled children, learning a new code (cursive) comes with great difficulty.
- Encourage the use of the computer with word processor for children whose writing is slow and labored. The machine acts as a sequencer and "concretizer." This is particularly useful for the middle school and high school student who, because of motor or expressive language problems, finds writing slow and mistake prone.
- When the student is writing something new, encourage him or her to verbalize the response at the same time.
- When introducing new or distracting words, use color cues like a green letter at the beginning or the word and a red letter at the end of the word.
- The speed of mentation (processing mental information) is different in learning-disabled children. The teacher should make allowances by using "slow talk" and short sentences, and

by giving the learning-disabled child extra time to formulate his ideas.

- Children with learning disabilities don't "hear" (process) group directions well; it may save time to go directly to this child and repeat directions.

- One language skill deficiency is the disparity between the ability to recite orally as compared with putting information down in writing. Since nearly all regular school testing involves written work, children with this form of "graphic aphasia" underachieve in ordinary examinations since they cannot express in writing the information they have learned. It may be necessary to permit oral examination for these children.

- The teacher should find the child's true functioning level in reading, math, etc., and should be aware when assignments actually are over his head.

- Select special material for his reading alone. This should be gauged to give 90 percent success (and enjoyment). If a fifth-grade child can read at only the second-grade level, it is quite impossible for him to keep up and behave when he can decode only 40 percent of the words. High-interest, low-vocabulary material is needed for his solo reading.

- For reading grade-level material, a volunteer or family member is needed. This is essential if he is to keep up with his class in content of material. Most of these learning-disabled children can learn content (as opposed to basic skills).

- When the child is reading aloud, the difficult words should be supplied fairly quickly by the tutor so the child will get the story and enjoy it. It helps the tutor to realize that providing him a word on line five will not at all ensure his recognizing it on line ten. In fact, the child may recall it successfully on line thirteen and miss it again on the next page. This is typical with these children. It takes months, where the non-learning-disabled child takes days. Being forewarned is being able to avoid impatience and irritation.

- Recordings of the textbooks and lessons may be made by volunteers so the student can replay them at his or her convenience. Many children profit by reading silently along with the tape.

3. Permit simple classroom adjustments that will aid the child's efficiency and effectiveness.

- Review materials previously learned as often as possible until responses become automatic.
- When teaching a new concept, be sure, if possible, to illustrate the concept when giving a verbal explanation of it.
- When giving either oral or written assignments, do not give more directions than the student is able to cope with. For example, in a three-part assignment, it would be better to divide it and give directions for each part separately than to give all directions at once. As with all other suggestions in this section, this will depend on the capabilities of the student.
- When asking the student to respond to oral questions, give him plenty of time to answer. One study showed that the average time a teacher allows for a student to answer is about two to three seconds. Allow at least ten seconds, if needed. In some cases a half minute may be more appropriate.
- Provide a sheltered learning place for the child, freer from distractions; appropriate desk placement; use of movable partition—the private office idea.
- Help him to organize his study space. For example, he should have paper, pencils, crayons, and books in order and available for use, yet not in the way.
- Break his work into short segments. Place a paper over distracting pictures.
- These children can't suppress their reactions to these things, so they experience quick mental fatigue.
- Raise the "stimulus value" of elements to be learned. Any novel emphasis will help: color coding, emphatic use of voice, animation.

Specific Teaching Techniques

There are as many ways to teach as there are teachers. Through experience and research, numerous specialized techniques and programs for teaching the hard-to-teach child have been developed.

This is not the place to evaluate or to recommend specific methods; I am not a teacher and respect the unique training and experience they receive. Therefore, I have not dealt with specific remediation techniques in this chapter. Rather, I am speaking as an expert in child development attempting to point out methods that are developmentally appropriate for certain children with developmentally based disorders.

I strongly feel that the learning-disabled child deserves everyone's best efforts. All can learn if the right combination can be found. This often will require thorough diagnostic evaluation to determine the child's strengths and weaknesses. Then an informed search can be made for the best teaching techniques. Often a trial of diagnostic teaching by an experienced teacher will be the most effective means of finding the keys that unlock a learning disabled child's hidden potential.

The Importance of Reinforcement in the Learning Process

We hear, see, and feel things that are kept in our awareness for a short period of time and then forgotten. These things are not really learned. In order for a stimulus to be committed to the long-term memory and therefore learned, reinforcement must occur. Reinforcement is the process by which our conscious and unconscious mind is given a reason, or motivation, for committing a stimulus, thought, or concept to long-term memory.

Reinforcement is a complex and highly varied process. One of the most significant reinforcers for children is the internal, built-in drive to learn so characteristic of all children. Children innately want to learn about their world. A high percentage of all stimuli impinging on their senses is assimilated and committed to long-term memory (i.e., learned). This innate drive to learn persists in children until it is turned off by some negative reinforcement.

Negative reinforcement occurs when learning is made unrewarding, unpleasant, boring, or anxiety provoking. Under such circumstances, a child may begin to lose his internal motivation. For instance, the young child eagerly wants to talk with his parents and others about all the exciting things he is learning—that the tree is tall, the sky is blue, and bugs crawl. If his enthusiasm is met with continual indifference, he eventually will grow less interested himself in learning. The first grader is usually ready to learn to read. But if he finds the effort confusing and frustrating and finds he is not making progress, learning to read becomes unrewarding, and he eventually will quit trying.

The human mind has fantastic potential for learning, absorbing facts, and making leaps into new concepts. Each child has this innate drive to learn from the time his eyes begin to explore the environment, to his reaching for a rattle, to taking his first step, to saying that first word, to exploring the world of physics. This internal reinforcer, to remain strong, needs to be supplemented with external reinforcement for maximum learning to occur. This external reinforcement may take many forms. Certainly among the most powerful reinforcers are the social ones, such as recognition, encouragement, and praise.

The knowledge that actions on his part will get him something he wants, such as more free time, treats, money, or participation in a special activity, is a strong reinforcer.

Rewards must be immediate and tangible to the child to be effective. We should reward each little step toward the right goal, not wait to give one big reward for total perfection. As learning is reinforced, the material becomes more and more indelibly imprinted on the conscious and subconscious mind of the child.

We should remember that the strongest reinforcer of all is success. *Success breeds success.* As the child is able to accomplish tasks and sense personal fulfillment, he wants to repeat this pleasant experience. Thus it is important to plan the learning-disabled child's curriculum so that he experiences academic, personal, and social success.

Summary

As we said earlier, children spend more time at school than anywhere else except the home. Much of the child's sense of self-worth, or lack thereof, is determined by what happens at school. For many children, school is the place where they experience success, achievement, and self-affirmation. We would hope that this could be true for all children. And it can be if the teacher, counselor, parent, and other caring professionals work together to make it so. I am convinced that the teacher is key to this whole process.

For Thought and Discussion

1. These ideas are simply listed as suggestions and thought generators.

2. Brainstorm. List as many additional instructional ideas as you can think of either as an individual or as a group:

Chapter Fifteen

Finding Help for Your Child

Getting Started

> "I can remember the first report card Jimmy brought home. I looked at it and nearly cried," Mary said. "I would have if Jimmy wasn't standing there looking at me."
>
> "I hope you can help me," she sighed. "Jimmy is failing, and I don't know what to do. I don't know if the problem is me, Jimmy, the school, or something else. I just want some help for him."

This mother is speaking for many parents. Like Jimmy, their child is not doing well in school, is not responding to discipline, or is not getting along with people. They hurt because their child hurts. They are confused; they do not know where to turn. They have dozens of questions with no answers.

Children fail, underachieve, and have behavior problems for many reasons.

Some are not developmentally ready for the demands of school. Others may have subtle physical disabilities that interfere with their performance in the classroom. Still others have specific learning disabilities that close channels of learning open to other children. Many others will have neurological and developmental disorders, such as ADHD, that interfere with their ability to concentrate and organize a learning task. Others many have emotional problems related to stresses in their life. Very seldom does a child fail because he or she is "lazy" or "doesn't want to learn."

Finding the Right Helper for Your Child

Parents are often confused about the role, responsibility, and expertise of the many different professionals with which they and their children come in contact. Let's look at some of these resource people and consider how they can help parents and children find solutions to developmental and learning problems.

The Classroom Teacher. Next to the parents, the teacher is one of the most important people in the child's life. During the school years, the teacher at any given time will likely spend as many waking hours with the child as the parents. By training and experience, a teacher should be equipped to see the child in the context of his peers and provide some insight into the degree and nature of a child's variation from developmental, academic, and behavioral norms. Thus the observations and insights of a good teacher can be invaluable to the parents and other helpers who will be working with the child.

The teacher's understanding of the child and his or her unique needs, as well as the ability to teach basic concepts, will have an indelible influence on any planned intervention. Thus the teacher plays a vital role in both evaluation and intervention. Unfortunately, many classroom teachers have had little training in understanding and instructing the child who cannot learn in traditional ways. Teachers themselves are often frustrated. When they do recognize the child's problem, they have difficulty coping with it in overcrowded classrooms. A good teacher is to be valued and appreciated.

Parents can expect the classroom teacher to see the failing child as "a child with a problem" rather than just a "problem child." The classroom teacher should know how to refer the child and his parents to the proper resources within the school system. And finally, he or she should have the patience to help the child as much as possible, within the limitations of the classroom, until the optimal remedial situation is found.

The School Principal and Counselor. The next stop for parents is likely to be the school principal or counselor. While most of these are caring professionals, they also may or may not be trained to deal with the learning-disabled or ADHD child and his or her special needs. At least, they should recognize the need for evaluation and know what resources exist within their own school system as well as in the community at large. Many school counselors have gained additional skills in evaluating children having problems in the classroom. They can administer educational diagnostic tests and formulate remedial plans. When necessary, they can refer the child for additional help.

The Physician. Early on the family is likely to approach their family physician or pediatrician for help. While the physician is not able to prescribe a quick fix to the problem, he can help in some definite ways.

The physician can perform a general physical examination in order to assess the child's general health and to make sure that there are no illnesses interfering with the child's abilities or stamina. He should examine the neurologic function by assessing sensory input, reflexes, coordination, activity, and attention level. He should be aware of the subtleties of ADHD and be able to assess these or refer to a specialist who can. Of course, if medication is indicated for any reason, the physician is the one to prescribe and supervise its administration.

As a professional who is trained to be interested in the total child, the pediatrician or family practitioner is in a unique position to help parents, schools, and other agencies see the child has a "whole person" and to consider all the diagnostic and treatment possibilities. And the physician is obligated to be a "child advocate" seeking the very best comprehensive care available for his patient.

At times the primary care physician may recommend consultation with a medical specialist, such as a neurologist or a developmental pediatrician.

The Psychologist. In evaluating an underachieving child, the psychologist is an important member of the team. A clinical psychologist does not focus only emotional disturbances but is also a highly skilled individual trained to evaluate a person's mental, emotional, academic, and behavioral strengths and weaknesses. Through interview, observation, and the administering of various psychological and academic tests, the psychologist obtains insight into how the child functions. In addition, the psychologist is trained in a variety of counseling skills to help families and teachers relate positively to the child in trouble.

A psychologist may be on the staff of the school and get involved with the child early after a problem is suspected. Well-trained psychologists can be found on the staff of child guidance centers as well as in private practice.

Other specialists. Occasionally, other specialists will be needed to evaluate specific problems. A speech therapist can evaluate and treat a speech problem if it exists. The speech therapist is also trained to evaluate many of the language functions involved in learning and provide specific language therapy. An occupational or physical therapist may be consulted when a child has motor problems. In situations where significant emotional problems exist, a psychiatrist, social worker, or other counselor may be needed.

What to Expect of the Professional

Misconceptions and prejudices on the part of both professionals and parents often block free communication and lead to misunderstandings. It is important for parents to realize that the professional, be she teacher, psychologist, or physician, is human. Each of these professionals has his or her strong and weak points. No one has all the answers.

There are certain things parents should expect from the professional:

1. The professional should be willing to listen to what you, the parents, have to say. Not only is this the kind thing to do, but such listening is also necessary for a proper evaluation of the child. From my years of experience, I have learned that it does not matter how sophisticated my tests with which to make a diagnosis, the observations of parents and teachers are key diagnostic tools.

2. Expect the professional to be somewhat puzzled and uncertain about the underachieving child. The honest ones will quickly assure you that they do not have all the answers.

3. Expect the professional to be willing to cooperate with others in and out of his field in order to get a total picture of your child's overall needs.

4. Expect him or her to "see you through your struggle." The competent professional will not try to snow you with his cure-all plan and then forget about you. He will not offer you a cure but will be willing to work with you over time to meet your child's needs as they arise.

The lack of adequate diagnostic facilities has created a vacuum of need. Now that learning disabilities have become a "hot issue" generating increasing concern among parents, many unscrupulous, as well as well-meaning but misguided, operators have rushed to the forefront. Too often they offer the impossible in the form of a cure but are able to deliver little in substantive help.

Be Wary

Be wary of the following:

1. Anyone offering a complete or quick cure. So far I have not found any quick fix for these developmental problems. Help is certainly available, but it involves time, effort, and cooperation of many people. When fad treatments are latched onto, time, as well as the family's money, is often wasted.

2. Anyone pushing a method of treatment not known to the school personnel, your physician, and other professionals in the community. You can be sure that your child's teacher, principal, and counselor, as well as your pediatrician, are interested in what the community has to offer. If there is someone or some program around that can help, one of these people you trust is likely to be aware of its existence. They are not likely to recommend a program that is worthless and expensive.

3. Anyone who pushes just one form of therapy. The strengths and weaknesses of each underachieving child are unique. No one treatment is a panacea for each of them. Most children will benefit from a variety of interventions—through special education, behavioral management, and maybe medical treatment. Most competent professionals will be open to any possibly effective technique.

What Do I Do When I Don't Know Where to Start?

First start close to home. Check with your school officials and family physician. If they cannot help, they can often direct you to those who can. You may also check with a child development clinic, child guidance center, or rehabilitation center if one exists in your community. Some localities have comprehensive evaluation clinics staffed by teams of competent professionals to help you. These may be associated with a university, medical school, or guidance center. If you are left up a blind alley, after looking into known local resources, you can write the LDA (Learning Disabilities Association) or CHAADD (Children with Attention Deficit Disorders). These organizations can provide literature and other information. (Check these out on the Internet.)

Summary

You don't have to live in frustration when your child needs help with learning and behavior problems. Many people are available to help you. If you don't find that help in one place, keep looking. Begin with those professionals you are most familiar with, such your physician and school personnel. Talk to other parents, and contact the state and local chapters of LDA and CHAADD. And remember that under the law, your local school has the obligation to stick with you until reasonable and effective ways of educating your child are found.

For Thought and Discussion

1. What are some possible resource people from whom you can seek advice and help? List names and addresses.

2. What are some resource organizations locally from which you can seek help? List names and addresses.